1st Edition

Elsevier's

FACULTY DEVELOPMENT

An Interactive Solution

Sonja Sheppard, M.Ed., PhD, R.N.
Associate Director for Nursing and Allied Health
Hartnell Community College
Salinas, California

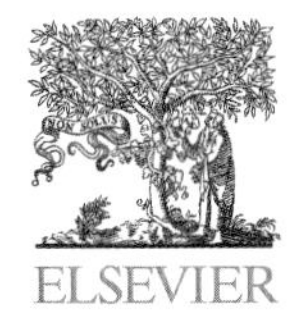

ELSEVIER

3251 Riverport Lane
St. Louis, Missouri 63043

ELSEVIER'S FACULTY DEVELOPMENT, FIRST EDITION
ISBN: 9780323722513

ISBN: 9780323722513

Senior Content Strategist: Linda Woodard
Director, Content Development: Laurie Gower
Senior Content Development Specialist: Rebecca Leenhouts
Publishing Services Manager: Shereen Jameel
Project Manager: Nadhiya Sekar
Design Direction: Bridget Hoette

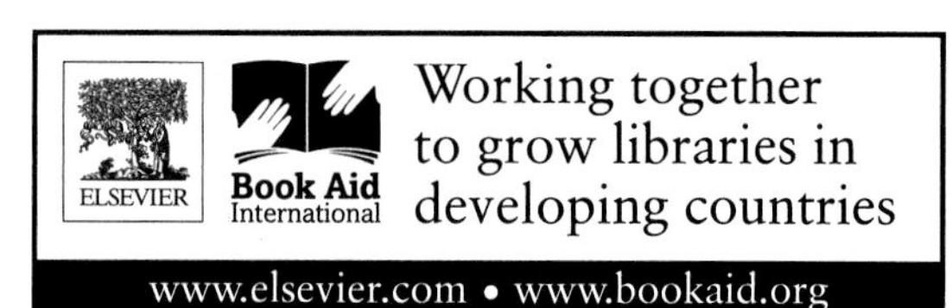

Printed in China
Last digit is the print number: 9 8 7 6 5 4 3 2 1

Elsevier's Faculty Development

Preface

Faculty are often hired for their knowledge but are not always the best or most experienced at teaching. Elsevier's Faculty Development will demonstrate ways you can be effective, engaging, and even have a little fun. Consider this worktext as a "quick how to" know your audience, assess their aptitude and learning styles, and meet their educational needs. As part of the learning process, you will do some soul searching to learn about your own strengths, passion, and expertise.

Designed for new faculty, this worktext is used in conjunction with the online course to provide a solid foundation to teach the teacher. It covers the basic tenets of education, particularly learning theories, learning styles, student engagement, assessments, and critical thinking. Additional chapters also offer ways to bridge the gap between various populations in the classroom and best practices for instruction. Background information is provided on various topics, with an opportunity to reflect, journal, and map out ideas. Each chapter goes into enough detail to cover the vast array of topics that new faculty are often challenged by. With various real-world examples, opportunities to write out ideas and questions, and some unconventional ideas to use in the classroom, it is designed to help faculty meet the modern needs of the student. Active learning for adult learners is the primary focus, as most college classrooms struggle with keeping students interested and able to persist in their courses.

This worktext is also helpful for other faculty who need fresh ideas or who have not had positive outcomes. As education continues to shift and student learning becomes more of the priority, faculty must keep up with this ever-changing swing. This worktext will help all faculty create more invigorating activities to facilitate learning and will inspire faculty to learn more themselves.

An accompanying online course reviews the concepts that you've learned in the worktext using engaging interactive exercises and case scenarios. Also included in the course is a **bonus module** that discusses best practices for teaching online–certainly a priority for many instructors today.

Using both the handbook and online course, new faculty members can work through the content at their own pace. *Elsevier's Faculty Development* contains everything needed to turn subject matter experts into master teachers committed to student success!

Contents

Chapter 1

Learning Theories

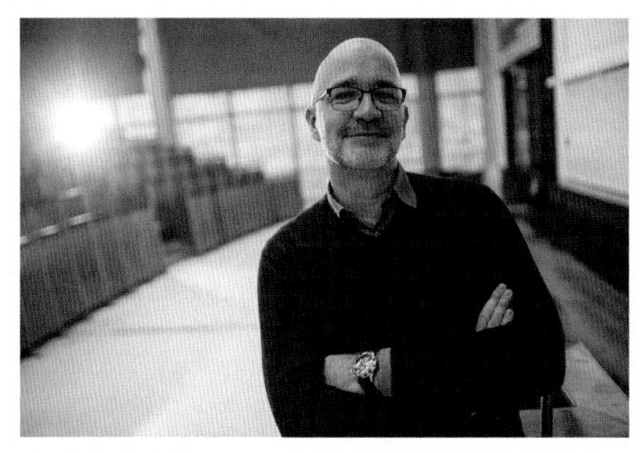

(AleksandarNakic/iStock.)

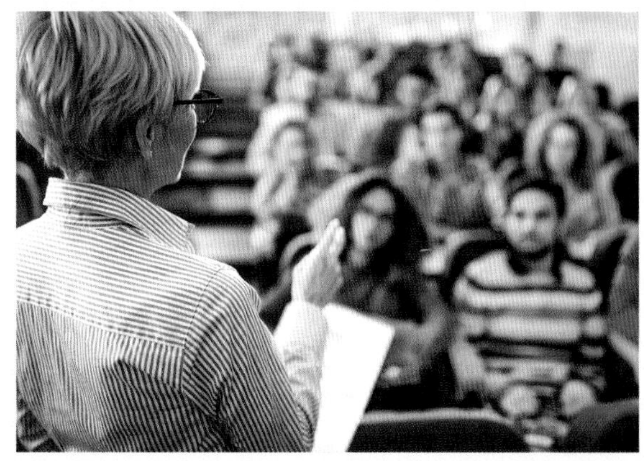

(skynesher/iStock.)

So, you want to be a teacher? Why? When did you get the calling, the gumption, the inspiration? Perhaps someone said you were good at explaining things, or you felt that you had so much knowledge you wanted it to share it with others. Perhaps there was an inner voice that drew you back to the classroom, or you felt it was time to give back to your community, or the next generation. Regardless of what brought you to the teaching profession, welcome! Teaching can be a very rewarding profession, but it can take a great deal of patience as you must first learn a few more things. While you are probably an expert in the subject you want to teach, not everyone knows how to share such knowledge with others. Even those who have gone through formal education and have studied teaching must continuously learn how to teach, as the pool of learners continues to evolve and teachers must keep up with this evolution in order to become successful in teaching.

Think back on how you were taught in high school, college, or even graduate school. Did you sit and listen to your professor who was at the whiteboard/chalkboard writing main points or showing PowerPoint slides? Were you actively engaged in class, answering questions, working in small groups? Did you find the lectures interesting or boring? Did you listen in class, but later teach yourself the key points in the material? When you think back on how you were taught, does it inspire you to teach that way, or the exact opposite? One of the most important aspects in teaching is to realize what works for *your* students, regardless of whether or not it worked for you.

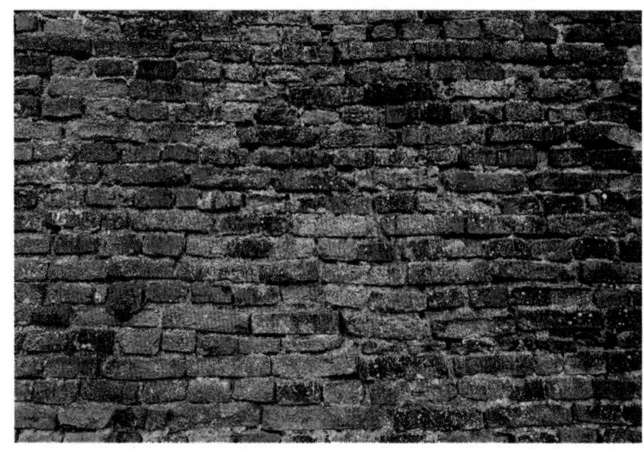

Fig. 1-1 (natasaadzic/iStock.)

Look at the photo in Fig. 1-1. What do you see—various colors, an image, perhaps a person, a dog, or maybe even nothing at all? Do you see it as three dimensional (3-D) or simply as a flat image? In looking at this image, many people will see different faces, colors, structures, and images. This is based on our perception, our eyesight/vision, and our interest. Learning is very similar to looking at this picture; based on our perceptions and interest, as well as other skills we may have, we will see things differently. Just as we see things differently, we learn differently. There is no right way to learn, and therefore there is no right way to teach (and there is no answer to what this image is; it is simply based on your perception). Though there is no right way to teach, the most effective way to teach is in the style that fits your class. As simple as that sounds, it is not simple at all. Undoubtedly your class will be made up of a variety of students—different ages, diverse ethnicities/cultures, all genders, and various interest levels. While some are very motivated and committed to the learning process, others are not as engaged or dedicated on their own.

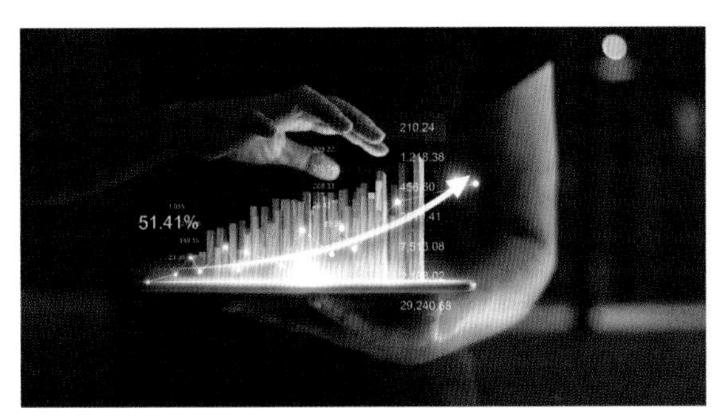

(ipopba/iStock.)

Often faculty believe that the information they have to present is so compelling and interesting that, of course, all students would want to listen, or because a student needs this class in order to graduate, they are obligated to listen and participate. Neither of these could be further from the truth. While there may be a very small population of students who will put forth the effort to listen no matter what, most students will follow along based on their own interest, perceptions, and motivation. Realizing this up front can decrease some of the frustration in teaching and guide the new teacher into a more rewarding experience. Education has shifted over the past few years; instruction is given in a multitude of settings and platforms, content is delivered electronically via simulation and virtual reality, and some courses are taught without even using a textbook. In order to keep up with this dynamic swing, teachers need to be willing to adapt and meet the needs of the students where they learn best. One way to help discover how to do this is by reviewing the theories that have influenced teaching and have provided a foundation in which to grow and build.

An Overview of Learning Theories

Why do we need to review learning theories? Understanding learning theories is important in order to guide teaching. If we, as teachers, regardless of our experience or education, fail to recognize how our students learn, we will struggle to keep them engaged, fall short of a positive experience (for them and us), and might very well feel frustrated and burn out quickly. Teaching is as much of an art as it is a science; as it evolves, it builds on prior experience and creates a broader space to generate more knowledge. Indeed, there is plenty of scientific research to support effective teaching strategies, based on learning theories and learning styles, yet there is no "one size fits all approach" to effective teaching. Great teachers, those most effective in helping students learn and actually enjoy their learning experience, find that they must pull from a variety of learning theories in order to adjust and adapt to their audience. When you consider the audience, your students, and how they learn, you will be able to be more objective about your own teaching and be able to make the necessary changes in your approach.

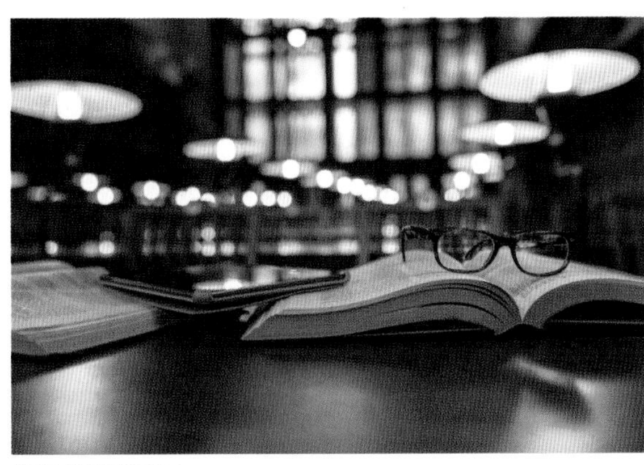

(Tashi-Delek/iStock.)

Learning theories have evolved into more expansive theories and have become more intertwined with one another. This makes it a bit easier to confront the modern classroom. As stated, there is no one right way to teach; none of the learning theories are more important, prevalent, or preferred over others. In fact, one approach may work with one class, but not another. Some students may be more receptive to rewards and consequences, while another student may not care about rewards at all, but rather be able to impart their own experience, ask questions, and be in charge of their own learning; you may even find all of the above in the same classroom! It is helpful for the new teacher, especially, to not take a rigid approach to teaching, based on any one idea or presumptive plan or theory. Teachers who ascribe to a variety of approaches to teaching and learning theories, and are flexible in their own delivery, will find their job most rewarding as their students will achieve a greater learning experience.

The Five Main Learning Theories

There are various theories related to how we learn. While we are not going to delve deeply into each one (that is saved for the master's in education class), we will briefly review the five pivotal theories that have been most instrumental in education: behaviorism, cognitivism, constructivism, humanism, and social learning. These are the primary theories when it comes to how people learn; together and individually, these theories have created a foundation in which all other theories related to learning have evolved. If you are keenly interested in learning theories, and want to study it more, know that there are many more theories and more information on each of these. Being that these are *theories*, they are based on one person's perception or idea, despite their research they simply offer another way of looking at learning.

Behaviorism

One of the oldest theories is behaviorism, which started with John B. Watson in 1913. Many of you might recall the study of Pavlov's dog, an exercise in classical conditioning whereby Pavlov would ring a bell and present food, stimulating the dog's appetite; the dog, anxious to eat, would begin to salivate. Pavlov was eventually able to condition the dog to salivate by simply ringing the bell. Conditioning and behaviorism were made popular in the 1960s with the research and works of B.F. Skinner. Skinner believed that the impetus behind our actions is learned; there is a reward or consequence that dictates how we respond, and thus, whether learning has taken place. No innate characteristic remains with us as we mature, but rather an ongoing process of trial and error.

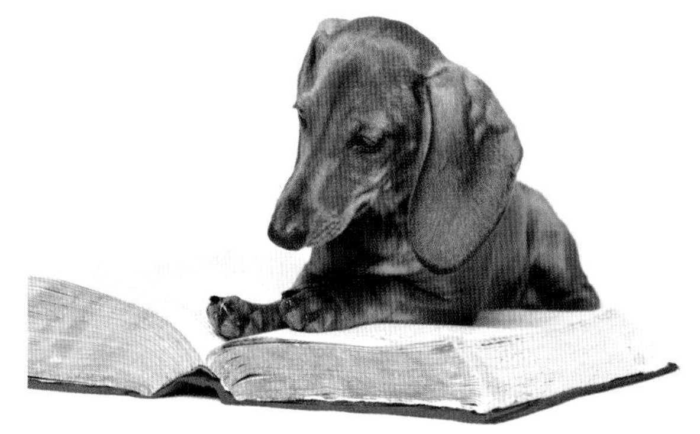

(Vladimirs/iStock.)

Behaviorism doesn't focus so much on motivation, but rather positive and negative consequences. While this form of conditioning works well with simple cause and effect material, it omits the introspection that is often needed in higher order thinking. In fact, when considering intelligence, emotions, and affect, behaviorists believe that these simply stem from genetics or from habit. While it may seem cold to consider learning to be so cut and dried, we often use this technique in standard classrooms. For example, gold stars are an example of positive reinforcement—when students receive a gold star for performing a behavior, they are being reinforced to repeat the behavior. While there is nothing wrong with earning a gold star, it will not necessarily be attractive to all students. Moreover, it is not based on any learning per se, but rather rewarding a desired behavior. On the flip side, negative reinforcement reinforces a behavior that avoids or removes a negative outcome. If you lock the door when students arrive late (and thus they must wait until break or go to the president's office), most students will arrive early or on time to avoid the embarrassment of being locked out. Other examples of behaviorism in the classroom include having students stay seated, raising their hand to ask questions, and adhering to a structured format. In a more pragmatic example, students in a skill-based program often need to demonstrate certain competencies, such as in health care vocations. If they do the task wrong, the teacher will correct them and continue to provide positive feedback until they perform the skill or task correctly. In each of these examples the student is not advancing their learning, but rather changing their behavior. The behaviorist theory focuses strictly on the desired outcome and uses various tactics to achieve the outcome. Tactics based on behaviorism can also be quite useful in classroom management which is explored further in Chapter 3. While it can be used with some effectiveness, faculty should be aware of college policies and department guidelines related to behavior as such tactics have come under scrutiny in recent years.

Cognitivism

In contrast to behaviorism, which focuses primarily on stimuli and responses, cognitivism relies on the inner working of the brain and processes such as memory (both short—and long-term memory). One of the most widely noted examples of memory and constructivism is Miller's notion that we can remember seven numbers (±2). Think about your social security number (nine digits), or your phone number (seven digits, without the area code); most driver's licenses are likewise five to seven digits. Cognitivism focuses on the brain and its various components, as well as how they work together, like a computer. Computers utilize memory, various functions, and required operations for them to work using each of these in a particular manner can produce similar outcomes. You don't have to know anything more about a computer other than: turn it on, wait for it to boot up, and find your desired browser. Regardless of the type of computer it is, they all have similarities in regard to operating systems, storage, and access of information (recall). For cognitive learning, the focus is on how to process the information, which can be done a variety of ways such as problem solving, being actively engaged, and using both internal and external factors to enhance learning. Activities that illustrate cognitivism include memory games, note taking, self-reflection, and small group discussions. The instructor is there as a guide, offering feedback, and as a facilitator, asking questions and promoting critical thinking in the learner. Consider a class on nutrition, whereby the instructor is there imparting their expert knowledge. Later, students may create a diet plan for a particular case, or debate which current fad diets are better for someone wanting to lose weight. The student is required to use their understanding of what they learned and process it to create a higher level of critical thinking.

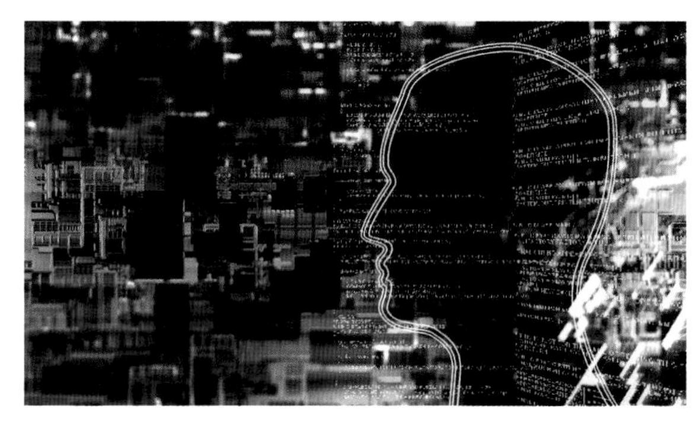

(MF3d/iStock.)

According to cognitivism, there are also various stages of development—whether in the young child (as with Piaget's studies) or in our psychosocial development (as with Erikson's stages of development). Based on where we are biologically, as well as in our formative development, we manifest different stages of development. Noting these developmental stages has influenced how we interact with people of all ages; they are widely used in such professions as health care, social work, and education. This development also feeds into our social, moral, and emotional development, which will most likely play a large part in your students' learning, and in how you teach. Your classroom may have a blend of recently graduated high schoolers, who are trying to establish their identity, be seen as competent, and become clear on their role as an adult, mixed in with older adults, who are more mature and well formed in their identity but unsure of being back in the classroom. Each of these students may have some doubts about their learning capability as they are in a sea of the unknown accompanied by different types of learners, a new environment, and most likely a unique approach to learning. Understanding the neurobiological aspect of cognitivism reminds us that we must include these developmental parts in viewing the whole student.

Constructivism

One of the more recent theories is constructivism, based on the works of such notable theorists as Piaget and Vygotsky. (It is important to note that Piaget, while contributing his research on cognitive development, was a constructivist.) Constructivism focuses more on the learner *constructing* their own learning from their surrounding environment and personal experiences, not necessarily from the instructor. Constructivism encourages the learner to build on prior knowledge and adapt their learning using invention, discovery, and creative questioning. While it is understood that learning doesn't occur in a vacuum, constructivism is a very active learning theory whereby the learner is at the helm. This is becoming more paramount as learners are entering a digital age, an age whereby their "environment" expands beyond the classroom, their circle of friends and family, and even their own community. Constructivism encourages such worldly exploration and social interaction in order to use the learner's baseline understanding of things to build on and expand into a greater understanding. Because traditional learners are digital natives (they were born into the digital age of cell phones, the Internet, and technology), they are often more comfortable with using such technology to construct more ideas and develop additional information. Nontraditional students and many faculty are considered digital immigrants, indicating that they did not grow up in such an environment but rather had to learn this foreign language and culture. This is important to realize as constructivism must allow the student to learn where they are, based on the tools they are most comfortable with.

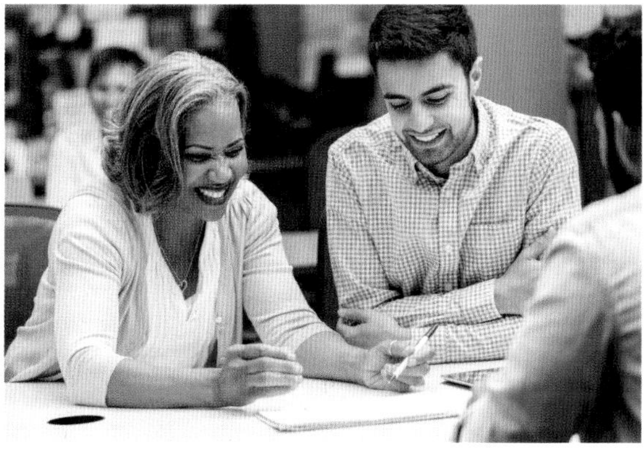

(SDI Productions/iStock.)

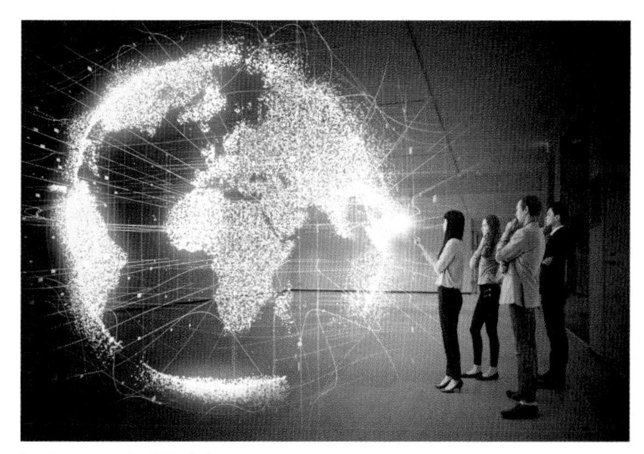

(metamorworks/iStock.)

Considering a class mixed with both traditional and nontraditional students, you may capitalize on this theory by pairing younger students with older students who have had more life experiences. These nontraditional or older students often have work or life experiences to draw upon that can assist their younger counterparts. Many skills learned from previous working environments or from various situations in life can offer a different perspective and are often transferable to the subject at hand.

Humanism

Looking at the whole person, their past and where they are presently, brings us to our fourth theory: humanism. Humanism emerged in the 1960s, which further focused on the learner as a whole person, instead of one who responds to stimuli or who has a mind of their own. In the humanism theory, faculty can better enable learners to reach their goals based on internal qualities, such as personal motivation. Humanism looks to the individual learner to be directed in their desire to learn, as well as modulate and self-evaluate their learning progress. According to this theory, learners are driven by what they want or need to know, guided by their emotional and intellectual abilities. Faculty, according to humanism, should create an environment that focuses on the learner's feelings, morals, and values, and what the learner needs in order to reach their full potential. Moreover, faculty must look to the individual learner, not the classroom as a whole. The uniqueness of the individual student is the focus; activities are geared toward expanding on each student's strengths and bridging the gaps in areas where students may not know material. This can be quite challenging in a large classroom, where there is great diversity; however, the instructor will find commonalties among the students and can still offer individual attention as needed.

Maslow's Hierarchy of Needs

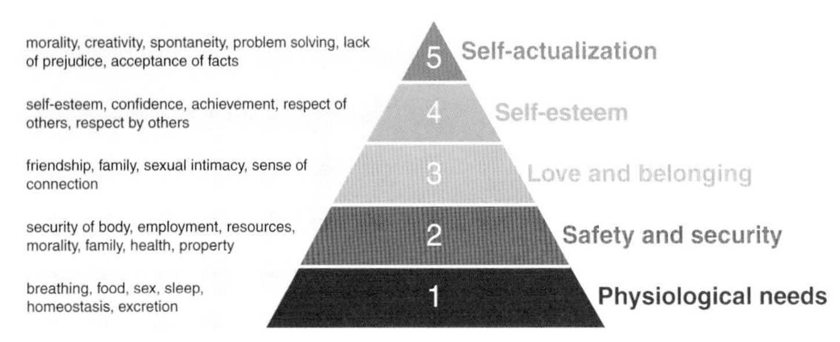

(PytyCzech/iStock.com.)

Theorists most known for their work in humanism include Maslow, Rogers, and Erikson (previously referred to regarding psychosocial development). Most health care and social service careers will introduce Maslow's hierarchy of needs as a pillar of human understanding. This hierarchy shows our needs as humans, starting with the basic needs of food, clothing, and other biological needs. Once these needs are met, we seek safety, security, and our need to feel protected. The third level of need is a sense of belonging, where our social connection takes place. We need to know we are part of a family, a community, a group of like-minded people. These three levels will be prominent in higher education, as your students should have their basic needs met, as well as their safety and a sense of belonging being that they are adults. However, keep in mind that if your student(s) struggle with these three levels it may be difficult for them to form solid relationships or achieve a sense of accomplishment. The fourth level seeks to find self-esteem through validation, a sense of appreciation and recognition. As you can imagine, if you are a homeless student and don't know where your next meal will come from, or where you will spend the night, a sense of accomplishment may not be your number one priority.

The fifth level is self-actualization, a sense of our purpose in life and knowing we are fulfilling our potential. Maslow's belief was that we all strive for self-actualization, regardless of whether we ever attain it; in fact, self-actualization is a state of being, not an end destination or a completion of self. In self-actualization you become your best; that is your overall goal, regardless of what other objectives might parlay into this goal. Those who strive for or achieve self-actualization have a connection with a bigger picture of their work and of themselves. They are often independent but humble; they work to improve areas in humanity but are very solitary. Various researchers believe that there have been those who have attained self-actualization, such as Mother Teresa, Albert Einstein, Buddha, and Abraham Lincoln. Others feel that self-actualization is actually never reached, but rather the elusive desire of all.

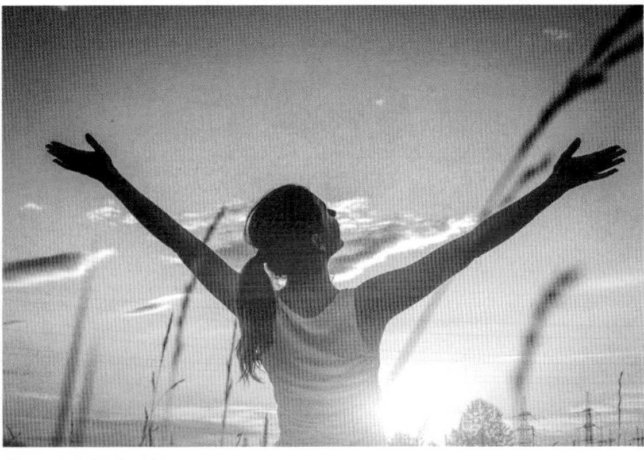

(Maryviolet/iStock.)

Though these five levels are well known, Maslow did have a sixth level, self-transcendence, which was published after his death in 1970. In self-transcendence we go beyond our own best person to provide a more global, albeit even more than mere human, sense of betterment for others. This notion is also part of various Eastern religions where we strive to be one with a universe and continuously better ourselves for a purpose greater than our self. The aforementioned people might also have reached this level, as their work benefited others globally and through various generations. Maslow's work has been used in many aspects of teaching, education, and research. It has also been translated into use in the workplace, to focus on inward, personal development needs; career needs; and the needs of the industry.

Social Learning

Social learning, the most recent learning theory, combines both cognitive and behaviorism with respect to one's cognitive abilities, personal environment, and one's own motivation. Bandura, most credited with this theory, initially looked at social learning as a form of modeling behavior. This is commonly seen in classrooms whereby the teacher provides instruction by performing a task or demonstrating a skill. Students can bring in prior knowledge of this task/skill or behavior and assimilate new information to expand on. Observation is crucial as the student will be required to replicate this new task/skill or behavior afterward. One current technique that emulates this is the flipped classroom. Students build on what they have witnessed from their instructor regarding how to lecture; then, by working in small groups, they are able to utilize one another's strengths and knowledge to present information to their peers and mimic this form of lecture. Again, the instructor is there to guide and offer feedback, but the onus is on the group to "teach" their peers.

Bandura eventually shifted this theory to encompass more of the individual's self-perception, their ability to evaluate self, and the ability to monitor one's self in order to achieve their desired goals. Social learning later became known as social cognition theory; coupled with this theory was self-efficacy, the belief a person is able to achieve their goals or a task. Self-efficacy, also credited with the works of Bandura, has become widely used in academia as it focuses on internal and external motivation, thereby incorporating many of the aforementioned theories. A good example of social cognition goes back to that gold star: if the student does not care about gold stars (or in the negative consequence, being locked out of the classroom), they will not change their behavior. Being that teachers struggle with keeping students attentive and engaged, it is important to accept the fact that students must not only be interested in receiving such information, but also believe they are capable of doing the work necessary. This is where self-efficacy plays a key role. If a student feels they are inept at doing the task required to earn the star, it will be very difficult to motivate them or keep them interested long enough to attempt the task.

Adult Learning

While the previous sections cover the five basic learning theories, there are other theories that influence instruction in higher education, primarily adult learning. Adults learn differently than children do, even if some of the techniques are the same. With adults, they have already had some education and have mastered some techniques; they come to the table with their own set of expectations and have a need to know more. We, as faculty, must honor this and tailor our instruction to include such things as the learner's concept of self, their prior experiences and knowledge, and what motivates them to learn. We must take into account that they have a more formal sense of their goals and want cooperation from the faculty member in achieving these goals. While all learning theories can be used with adult learners, the faculty must be clear on what the adult learner wants to learn and the style that works best with the student, the material being presented, and the environment in which you will be teaching. Included in this formula are the time constraints, as you will often have less time to expand and explore on complicated topics despite utilizing various creative techniques.

Malcolm Knowles was the first to research how adults learn and is credited with concept of adult learning, called andragogy (vs. pedagogy, which is how children learn). Realizing that adults learn differently, have different expectations and needs, and can participate more fully in their acquisition of knowledge, faculty can tailor their teaching to a more sophisticated process. However, this still requires foresight and planning, a topic we will discuss further in Chapter 2. Faculty must also incorporate motivation as a large influence in adult learning, as adults are motivated by a variety of both internal and extrinsic factors. When studying motivation there are as many theories surrounding motivation as there are surrounding learning; however, most of these can be summed up by realizing there are internal and external factors. Internal motivation is based on self-determination and the concept of efficacy (as previously mentioned with Bandura's self-efficacy in social cognition). This theory suggests that people achieve better results when they clearly know they can; their own belief in their skills and capability is far more important than simply the knowledge of the subject. Those with a higher self-efficacy therefore work harder to ensure they reach the goal of the task or of the learning objective, and can stay focused with the work at hand. Self-efficacy plays a role in goal setting, as it requires persistence and self-regulation, qualities which are part of the self-determination theory (otherwise known as SDT).

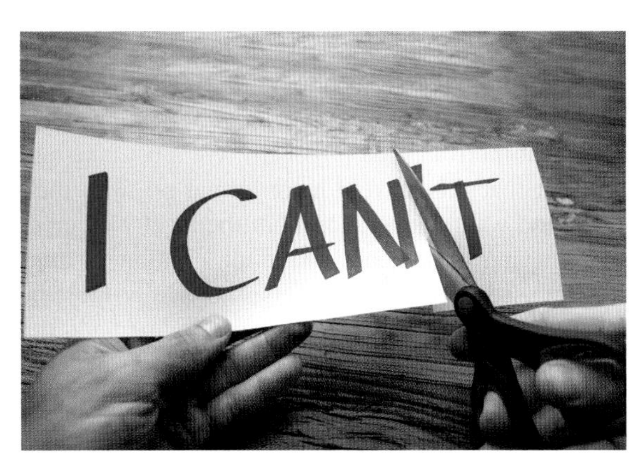

(AndreyPopov/iStock.)

Self-Determination Theory (SDT)

SDT postulates that we all have a need to feel autonomous, competent, and related. Being autonomous implies that students have a choice in their learning, and willfully want to learn. It also implies that students can stimulate their own motivation internally and thus increase their competency. In competency, the student becomes better at the task at hand and improves, which in turn reinforces their self-efficacy. If a student believes they can do a task, and then does it with great success, they prove that they can do it and this increases their belief in their skills. This cycle becomes a positive spiral and perpetuates itself continuously. As this cycle progresses, the student also must connect outside of themselves. Relatedness occurs when the student steps out of themselves and connects with others; as the student becomes more related to the people and the environment around them, their value and sense of efficacy continue to increase or improve. Again, the paralleling cycle of positive spins fuels their internal motivation. This internal or intrinsic motivation provides enjoyment for the keen student; no longer does the task seem to require as much effort, or at least, the effort is not considered in a negative fashion. Their enjoyment of the task enables them to continue the task, regardless of how arduous it might be. As a teacher, it is important to identify students who possess such intrinsic motivation; we want to feed this motivation as much as we can, or at least create the environment in which it feeds itself. We want that positive cycle to continue spinning as it will unite and ignite other students' motivation.

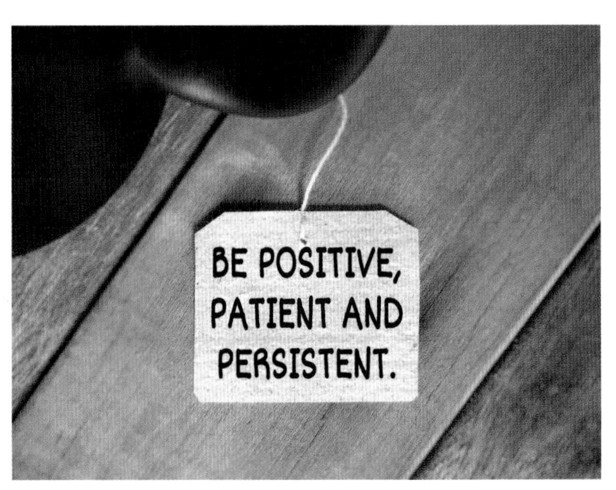

(Coompia77/iStock.)

Internal and External Motivation

While many adult students have intrinsic motivation, others will need external rewards to maintain their motivation. External motivation can be seen in a wide range of behaviors, such as accolades or praise, grades, or even an actual physical reward such as a certificate, trophy, or medal. These rewards must be of value to the student who needs such external motivation to compel them to persist. If the reward is meaningless or has no value to the student, the benefit is lost and can devalue the educational experience. Take for example a student who thrives on acquiring public praise and needs some tangible connection to this praise, such as a medal or certificate. If you simply gave them a high five for their achievement, or if the certificate was mailed to them, it would not be as effective in motivating the student. However, if you provided the certificate at the beginning of class (in front of their peers), or at a ceremony, and outwardly praised the student for their achievement, it would have more meaning and thus motivate the student to work harder and persist in their educational journey.

There has been a great deal of research as to whether external factors influence internal motivation; however, for the purposes of this chapter we will accept the fact that gold stars, praise (often referred to as atta-girl or atta-boy), and an occasional high five stimulate internal motivation or at the very least, provide external motivation. While you may not be able to do a complete history of each student and understand how they are individually motivated, you will begin to notice changes when you provide praise and connect with students on an individual basis. This connection to students is especially helpful as you learn more about how to reach them, for that can provide the map on how to teach them. When a student beams after receiving praise for their presentation, or when you ask a student to lead a particular discussion and they perform with precision and professionalism, you also show that you can individualize your efforts to meet the needs of your students. This talent requires great sensitivity, time, and a sincere desire to connect with and serve your students.

Knowing how to motivate students, or where their motivation comes from, has rewards for the faculty as well as the student. When students stick with their learning process long enough to reach their goals, for both short and long term, the faculty gain a sense of pride and value. Likewise, knowing that amotivation exists among students allows faculty to not put so much pressure on themselves if a particular subject or exercise is not received with the same amount of zeal and zest spent on creating it. Many of the first few lectures and class activities will be a trial and error for the faculty and for the students who are not familiar with active learning. If you started the first day of class by asking "what motivates you," you will get myriad answers, and some may not even be accurate. Students may not realize what motivates them on an inner level, or that they have permission *not* to be motivated. After a series of class days, this self-reflection on the student's part may be entertained, especially after a few trial and errors. A later conversation that asks the student to consider what keeps them on track is likely to yield more accurate answers, as both you and the student have had a chance to give and receive feedback. A student may tell you that they really don't care for the high praises in class but do appreciate your one-to-one time tutoring them.

Recent research on SDT adds two additional components to this theory: the concept of one's welfare (mental and physical health) and the ability to thrive. In addition to being autonomous, connected, and related, a person must have a positive sense of their own well-being and believe that they can flourish. These two additional components bring a higher level of one's self so that it incorporates a deeper awareness of one's capacity. Much like Maslow's hierarchy of needs, the student must be able to attend to these various components and reinforce them, as well as regulate their usefulness. While much research in education has been based on SDT, other theories on motivation that parallel SDT include Vroom's expectancy theory (which postulates there is a direct connection between one's effort and their performance), Zimmerman's theory on self-regulation (also tied in with self-reflection and performance), Eccles's theory of expectancy-value (which correlates the value of the task with one's self-efficacy), Weiner's theory of attribution (a 3-D approach to motivation that includes locus, stability, and control), and Csikszentmihalyi's theory of flow (comparable to what is called "being in the zone"—so engulfed in a pleasurable task that you are extremely focused). Within each of these theories is the interwoven aspect of motivation and the ability to perform based on an internal drive to succeed versus external rewards.

Each theory has validity in the teaching realm, and effective teachers will base their teaching on a variety of theories. While this was an abbreviated review of learning theories, it is important to realize that people learn differently, in a variety of settings, and can change or adapt based on their environment, interest, and perceived need to learn. Whether or not you support one or more (or none) of these theories, you, as faculty, must be able to grasp ideas that are beyond your own comfort level and knowledge base. After all, you are not teaching to an audience of you! Whatever worked for you, or didn't work for you in your learning, does not necessarily equate to how your students learn. Even if you have taught previous classes, what worked with those students may not work with a new class. This is where teaching requires a bit of humility, flexibility, and openness to adjustments as needed. Effective instruction requires a greater focus on the learner, not necessarily the material being presented. By knowing your audience, the students, and how they learn, you can present the material in ways that will interest them and keep them engaged, as well as achieve the prescribed outcomes. In other words, you can be working smarter, not harder.

Learning Styles

Understanding learning theories can guide faculty to understand and embrace various learning styles. This is important as each person learns differently, in a variety of ways, and may not even know exactly how they learn most effectively. Just as there are various theories related to how we learn, there are also many different ideas on the styles or ways students learn. It was previously thought that there were simply three different learning styles: tactile, visual, and auditory; however, today's research indicates there are 70 different learning styles. Some of the more common theories and models include VARK's model (visual, auditory, reading/writing, and kinesthetic learning), Gardner's multiple intelligence theory (also known as MIT, which includes nine different intelligences and learning styles), and Kolb's experiential learning style theory (a four-stage learning process using diverging, assimilating, converging, and accommodating). It is important to understand that each of these is a theory, meaning none are "proven" to be the best way for students to learn. What they do offer is some insight into how we, as teachers, can present information to students in a variety of ways to reach a variety of students.

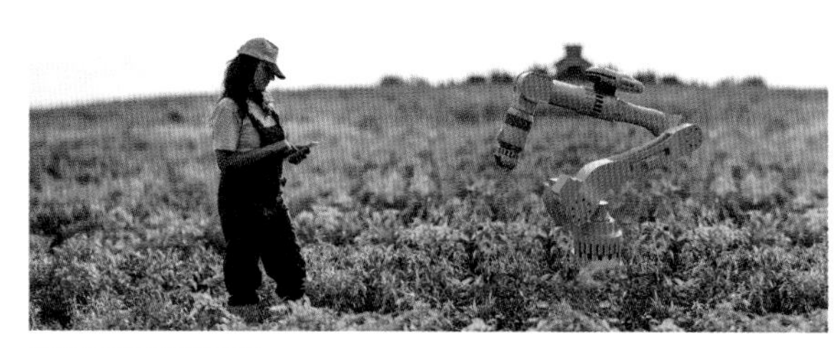

(baranozdemir/iStock.)

Multiple Intelligences

Coupled with learning styles is the capacity to learn, or intellect. Intellect, or intelligence, involves not only one's ability to learn, but also their ability to solve problems and understand the material. While it was previously thought that intellect could be measured based on a single test (such as an IQ test, originally developed by Binet), it has been discovered that there are other forms of intelligence, such as emotional intelligence (based on the works of Daniel Goleman), general and specific intelligence, and creative intelligence (based on the works of Sternberg). There is also some controversy that we have a variety of different, or multiple intelligences (based on the works of Howard Gardner). As previously mentioned, Gardner created the multiple intelligence theory or MIT, which claims that we are not bound to a single intelligence, but rather nine areas whereby a person may have higher aptitude:

- logical/mathematical—good with numbers, ability to think abstractly
- linguistic/verbal—good with words, speaking, verbal skills
- tactile/kinesthetic—good with hands-on skills, body movement

- aural/musical—good with rhythm, can hear different tones
- spatial/visual—able to "see" it in their mind, good with spatial abstract context
- intrapersonal/solitude—able to be self-aware, in tune with self
- interpersonal/social—in tune with others, empathetic
- naturalistic/environmental—good with plants, animals, and nature
- existential—deeper awareness of self and one's purpose in life

These areas also correlate with how students learn and can be used as a launchpad to ensure faculty touch on different teaching methods in order to reach a broader audience.

Because there are so many views on learning theories, intelligences, and learning styles, there are also various arguments on how to assess one's aptitude or intelligence. The Wechsler Adult Intelligence Scale (WAIS) is often used to assess adult's intelligence, as well as aptitude tests (such as the ACT, SAT, or GRE) for educational purposes. Many institutions may require an entrance exam prior to students being accepted into your program. However, regardless of how well or poorly students perform on these or any test, we must realize that this is only a snapshot of the person, and only captures how well they perform on that test. Researchers may not agree on any one specific test to evaluate the overall intelligence of a person, but they all agree that there are different ways to evaluate a person's ability to succeed. Furthermore, it is important to note that intelligence is not static—it can improve with additional learning. It is also influenced by both nature and nurture: areas such as one's diet, environment, socioeconomic factors, and students' genetic makeup can affect and change one's intelligence. With this information, it is important for the faculty member to realize the part they play in directing one's learning, and how their intellect will evolve based on their learning. This is not to say that each student's intellectual outcome is a result of the faculty member or their teaching style, but to stress the importance of including a variety of teaching styles that support learning.

To facilitate various learning theories and learning styles, there are a wide variety of resources to encourage active learning activities such as flipping the classroom, think/pair/share, minute papers, concept mapping, and peer teaching. Descriptions of these can be readily found on the Internet and can range from simple strategies (how do I keep students interested during the last 30 minutes of class), to full curricula based on student-led instruction. In Chapter 2 we will review planning, and in Chapter 4 we will review these engagement activities in more detail. However, it is important to keep in mind that these resource topics have a large range; it can easily overwhelm even the most seasoned faculty. Selecting one or two strategies and determining their effectiveness, as well as your comfort level, is a good way to start out. As mentioned, you will be continually adding new tools to your repertoire as you determine which techniques are better for your students, based on the material and time allotted for your course.

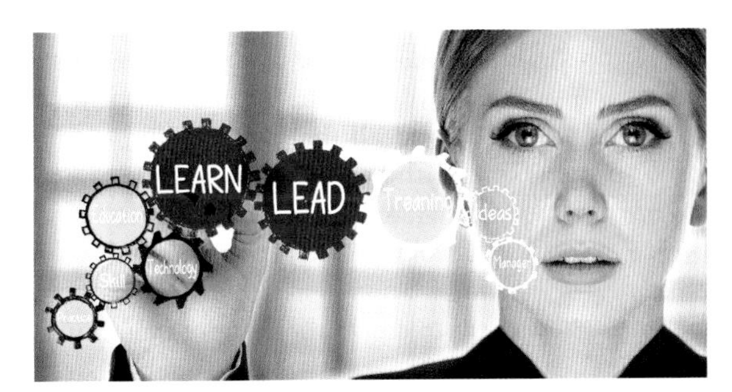

(guvendemir/iStock.)

Bloom's Taxonomy

One the most relevant tools in higher education is Bloom's taxonomy of learning. Though it has been revised, it is a staple in higher education as it shows the different levels of learning and what each level can be used for. When looking at this taxonomy, it is easy to see that the lowest level is the simplest to perform but it doesn't reach the higher order of thinking needed to meet all educational goals. When a student can create an original work, it is felt that they have learned the material and reached the objective.

Bloom's Taxonomy

create — Produce new or original work
design, assemble, construct, conjecture, develop, formulate, author, investigate

evaluate — Justify a stand or decision
appraise, argue, defend, judge, select, support, value, critique, weigh

analyze — Draw connections among ideas
differentiate, organize, relate, compare, contrast, distinguish, examine, experiment, question, test

apply — Use information in new situations
execute, implement, solve, use, demonstrate, interpret, operate, schedule, sketch

understand — Explain ideas or concepts
classify, describe, discuss, explain, identify, locate, recognize, report, select, translate

remember — Recall facts and basic concepts
define, duplicate, list, memorize, repeat, state

(Verishagen, N: Social Media: The Academic Library Perspective, 2019, Chandos Publishing, Canada.)

This taxonomy provides another opportunity to reflect on how you want to reach your goals and objectives. With each level of the taxonomy, other tools can be incorporated to help the teacher guide the student. For example, to enhance memory (remembering) we often use mnemonics, sing-song phrases, abbreviations, or acronyms to retain pieces of information. Later, the rhyme or acronym can easily be used to recall that information (think back to the colors of the rainbow—Roy G. Biv—or how you remember which months have 30 days and which have 31). Teachers can guide students with this type of learning for appropriate subject matters, but also allow them to create their own mnemonics. This can be appealing to a variety of students based on the subject material, their learning style, and the goal of instruction. This is where the instructor must be capable of sensing how their students learn and what is needed to fully grasp the material. While it may seem that all students should enjoy games and fun activities, some prefer a more logical approach. Due to the recent changes in education, our students come with a variety of backgrounds, interests, and expectations. Moreover, students are entering higher education at different times of their life; some are traditional, indicating they are recent high school graduates, others are nontraditional adult learners who have been out of school for a while. While some have had some work experience, many students are the first in the family to attend college and may have never worked.

The savvy teacher will understand all learning theories, styles, intelligences, and the taxonomy of learning; however, their course will be planned on what is best for their students. They will adopt new ideas, exchange ones that are ineffective, resurrect previously forgotten good ideas, and keep an open mind. While they may enjoy internal rewards with the satisfaction of teaching, they remain diligent in knowing their own strengths, where they need to grow, and can plan their own learning accordingly. These teachers remain humble, flexible, and grounded in the realization that indeed they are making a difference in the lives of their students. On the road to being this teacher, we will ask that you perform some activities yourself, including self-reflection (which may require some soul searching), journaling, and using the knowledge gained through this workbook and the online portion to answer some questions. You are free to use other resources, including your institution's assigned mentor, your personal and professional peers, and the Internet if you remain open and objective. Remember, there is no one way or right way to teach; you are well on your way toward learning the best way to teach your unique group of students.

Journal: Self-reflection

1 *Self-reflection: how I was taught*

In reviewing these theories, which one strikes a similar chord in how you have been taught? Which one is in alignment with how you will teach? Let's do a few exercises to pull this all together. Think back on some of your most favorite (and least favorite) courses, whether in grade school, high school, or college. What did you enjoy the most? The least? Which classes do you remember? What was significant about these classes? Jot a few notes here about your own previous learning.

2 *Learning theories*

Considering the course(s) you will most likely be teaching, think about the learning theories we reviewed. For each of these theories, write down one activity that supports that theory. Feel free to browse the Internet for ideas or speak with another seasoned faculty member about this.

a. Behaviorism:

b. Cognitivism:

c. Constructivism:

d. Humanism:

e. Social learning:

Additional notes:

3 *Motivational techniques for my class*

Before you run to the dollar store and stock up on brightly colored pencils or spend your first paycheck on gift cards before you ever get paid, consider some ideas that may be used as external rewards. As mentioned, students must find these rewards valuable in order for them to be effective. (Hint: most of the rewards cost nothing except compassion and foresight.) Also remember to check with your facility as there may be a budget limit to what you can offer, or policies regarding certificates, awards, and other acknowledgments. There may be campus-wide initiatives for these categories as well; it is important to be well versed or have the appropriate member of your department share how students can earn these awards to ensure they earn and receive them appropriately. Most students will start a portfolio early in college and look forward to adding these awards throughout their educational journey to share with employers.

a. Some tangible rewards I want to use:

b. Some intangible rewards I want to use include:

c. How will I assess what rewards will motivate my students?

d. How will I know if these rewards are effective?

4 *Using MIT in the classroom to create diverse experiences*

In reviewing the multiple intelligence theory, modern classes often include a variety of creative learning exercises to ensure you reach your students with their diverse learning styles. Considering your classes, and using Gardner's MIT classifications, write down how you would use each of the styles with your class. Note: do NOT use all nine on one class!

Some examples might be:

- *A class on dosage calculation*—use logical/mathematical and aural/musical (be specific in your exercises); allow extra time for hands on/tactile/kinesthetic if using actual equipment such as syringes.

- *An orientation class*—use interpersonal/social, linguistic/verbal, and existential (why did student join this class?); possibly naturalistic—go outside and interact with nature.
- *A class closer to graduation*—intrapersonal/solitude, visual/spatial (where does the graduate see themselves after graduation), and existential; be sure to allow time for journaling.

a. Logical/mathematical:

b. Linguistic/verbal:

c. Tactile/kinesthetic:

d. Aural/musical:

e. Spatial/ visual:

f. Intrapersonal/solitude:

g. Interpersonal/social:

h. Naturalistic/environmental:

i. Existential:

Additional notes:

5 *Bloom's taxonomy and my class*

Again, considering your upcoming class(es) that you will be teaching, look at each of the levels of Bloom's taxonomy. Write at least one exercise that students would do to demonstrate their knowledge of that level. This can be for the same course (at varying times) or different courses. Again, feel free to use Internet resources to spark ideas or jumpstart your own thinking.

a. Remember:

b. Understand:

c. Apply:

d. Analyze:

e. Evaluate:

f. Create:

Additional notes:

6 *Journal exercise*

Go back to the first paragraph of this chapter. Why *do* you want to be a teacher? How will you make a difference in the lives of others? Spend some time reflecting, as you will want to review this from time to time; it can rekindle your interest and passion when you feel overwhelmed. Answer the questions below honestly—this is simply for you to reflect on.

a. I want to be a teacher because:

b. I can make a difference in student's lives by:

c. What I want most out of my teaching experience is:

d. I will need help in teaching in these areas:

e. The person who can help me with this (item d) is:

f. The person who inspires me the most to be a good teacher is:

7 *Learning for the teacher*

Just as we discussed the learning theories, learning styles, and Maslow's hierarchy of needs with regard to your students, let's shift that focus to you. Answer the following questions honestly, based on you—your needs and desires. Again, this is a self-reflection exercise and doesn't have to be shared with anyone.

a. What rewards do you enjoy? This is outside of your salary or any bonus you may receive from your employer. Think about the external rewards, positive feedback from your boss, accolades from student surveys, or internal rewards such as personal growth or self-satisfaction in mastering a particular subject.

b. Which of the learning theories is most familiar to you, either in how you learn or how you have taught? Which one will be more of a challenge to use?

c. Considering the various learning styles and nine intelligences as defined by Gardner, which ones do you often use in learning? (If interested, there are informal online learning assessments that can help you identify these.) Which ones are not strengths for you? (This can indicate an area where you may need outside resources or spend more time exploring ways to use this style to meet the needs of your students who have different learning styles than you do.) Perhaps you are good with logical, verbal, social, and existential learning, but struggle with naturalistic (maybe you are not an outdoorsy person). Identify your strengths below:

d. How will you take those areas that need improvement to the next level, like the example of the naturalistic learning style mentioned above?

____

____

____

____

____

8 *While we have covered a great deal related to learning, perhaps there are some questions you still have. They may be outlined and even answered in future chapters, or they may be better explained through a mentor. It is important to write down your ideas, thoughts, fears, and concerns, whether or not they are addressed later, as they are important enough to occupy your mind now. Be sure to review these questions before the end of the teaching course and bring them up if they are not addressed in future chapters.*

____

____

____

____

____

____

____

____

____

____

____

____

____

Tell me and I forget.
Teach me and I remember.
Involve me and I learn.
Benjamin Franklin

Chapter 2

Course Planning

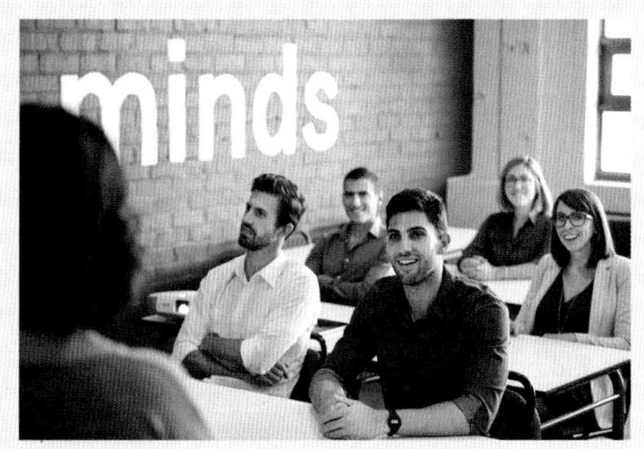

(AJ_Watt/iStock.)

In Chapter 1 we covered many fundamentals when it comes to learning. We reviewed the five major learning theories (behaviorism, cognitivism, constructivism, humanism, and social learning). Maslow's hierarchy of needs was also touched upon to remind us of how important it is that we understand our students' well-being: whether their basic needs are taken care of. It might be helpful to do a quick check in with your class to ensure students realize that having a good night's sleep, a healthy breakfast, and coming to class with an open mind are still important in college. We touched on motivation, both internal and external, while looking at self-determination and other theories that support motivation. Self-efficacy, or the belief that one has in themselves in performing the task, is a crucial part of motivation. We reviewed Bloom's taxonomy and realize that to get students to the higher order of thinking, we must ensure we offer the right combination of activities to stimulate them. All of this information in Chapter 1 gave us a platform on which to build; now, let's use that information to plan your course.

While it may seem that teaching is second nature, planning your course can be one of the most instrumental and decisive things you do to help yourself succeed. No doubt you know your material, may even be an expert at it, but how you relay that vast amount of knowledge to others can make a huge difference, and it doesn't come easily or by second nature. You have probably had the opportunity to teach others, perhaps your coworkers, peers, at a community class, or even other college classes; you may have had fewer formal opportunities, such as teaching your children or family members. These can help you, but learning how to teach the subject matter you are assigned requires a great deal of planning and focus. Consider it like charting a course on a map—you don't jump from where you are to the destination, you must plan out a path that is the most efficient, scenic, or direct route. Even with careful planning, your path may go off course or be zigzagged, but if you stay focused on your destination you will arrive.

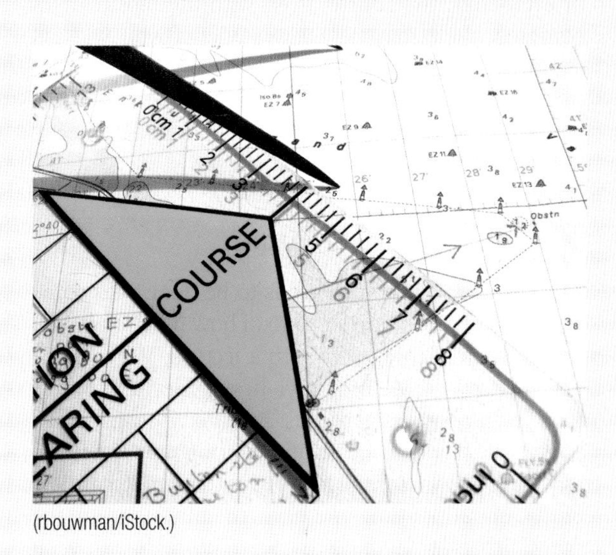

(rbouwman/iStock.)

Planning requires that you start with the end in mind and include a variety of activities to keep yourself and your students engaged. You may wonder what this means, as teaching is often seen as "me teach, you listen." This couldn't be further from the truth, as students are much more a part of the learning and thus the planning process than before. Our educational paradigm has shifted to being learner or student centered, and more of our focus is on the student; their goals, their style of learning, and ensuring they meet the outcomes. It is often said that prior planning prevents poor performance. When it comes to teaching, you need to take this to heart. Don't wing it—students will know the difference.

How to Plan

There are various exercises and activities at the end of this chapter that will guide you in course planning. Remember your course will not be static; it will evolve based on the needs of your students. Some things will work, some won't, some you will edit and use in a different way—regardless of what works and what doesn't, be flexible and be kind to yourself. Your students are the litmus test of your planning effectiveness; if they can meet the goals, objectives, and expectations of the course, the chances are your planning was spot on. However, this doesn't mean that all students will pass the course, or that everyone will earn an "A" or even enjoy the course. Even with the most careful planning, there may be a few students who will fall short of the expectations, not meet the goals or objectives, and may even drop out from the program. While it is helpful to evaluate this, it is more important not to take it as a direct result of your teaching.

What Do You Have to Teach?

Planning for your course needs to be done with some realism. There is no preset ratio of how much time you need to plan a course, or even a lecture. While some institutions offer 2 hours to 1 hour of lecture, others may be more or less generous. Based on how generous your institution/college is with granting prep time, you may have a few weeks or a few days to plan. Regardless of the amount of time you have, the questions are the same: What do you *have* to cover? What do you *want* to cover? Who is your audience? What activities do you want them to do? At the end of the day, what is most important? The first question regarding what you *have* to cover is based on the instructional or lesson plan; this plan (often called an IP or LP) is a list of preset goals and objectives identified by the institution/college. These goals are part of the curriculum which has been approved by various regulatory bodies, such as an accreditation agency, practicing board, or the college's Board of Trustees. Always confirm what leniency you have in carrying out the goals and objectives, as some institutions/colleges are rigid and faculty must adhere to the hours/days, while others allow flexibility whereby the goals and objectives can be met at any time within a semester. Once armed with this information, you will be sure to avoid having to rewrite your plan when the time comes to execute it.

Syllabus

In addition to the goals and objectives for this course, you will need a syllabus. Is there a preset syllabus, or will you create one? Your syllabus must be clearly written as it is your contract with your students; it has the goals and objectives for the course, as well as an overall (and perhaps detailed) view of the daily or weekly requirements. What textbooks and resources are being used? Are there whole chapters included or just a few pages from the text? Are there any outside reading or online resources students should be aware of? When are assignments due? When are the tests? What will the test cover (regarding chapters or other sources)? What is your attendance and late policy for submission? Are there any excused absences? Where do students go if they disagree with you and want to file a grievance? All this information should be listed in your syllabus, even if it is in your college's catalog. For online courses, or if an online syllabus is available, it is important to provide the link to the catalog to ensure that students have the most current policy.

When it comes to the syllabus and expectations, think of the syllabus as the "cheat sheet" for any faculty who might have to take over for you at the last minute. Despite the many hours of preparation you are doing for this course, if there was an emergency and you couldn't teach it, your syllabus (along with the IP) is there to guide the substitute faculty member. Having a detailed listing of all exams and quizzes, including the midterm and final exam, is crucial so that students know what to expect regarding assessments. In addition to the academic side of the syllabus, it is also a good idea to include other expectations, such as your office hours, where to go for tutoring, and your personal expectations of behavior (we will cover this in in more detail in Chapter 3). While some items may be listed in the college catalog or student handbook, you will want to reiterate them so your students have a focused spot when looking for information.

Tests and Quizzes

Once you know the goals and objectives, look at the tests, quizzes, and exams. These assessments will steer you and keep you on track and identify the areas you *want* to cover. There is an enormous difference between using these assessments to guide your course planning versus teaching to the test. Teaching to the test focuses only on test questions (and answers); it assumes the goal of the lecture is to ensure students are experts on the testing material. Such lectures lack endurance and fall short of reaching other goals, such as state licensure or national exams; therefore this practice is frowned upon and often grounds for dismissal. Instead of this practice, it is advisable to have assessments as guiding principles in addition to goals and objectives. These combined resources offer a blueprint which reveals the overall picture for the course; filling in the details is where creativity and expertise play their part. Consider the goals and objectives as a destination—how you get there is up to you.

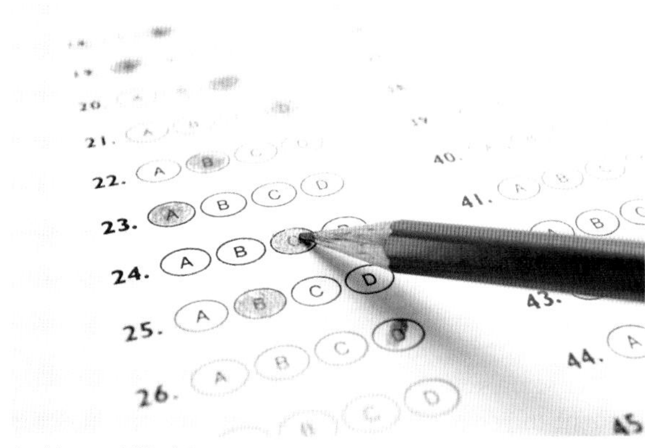

(sasirin pamai/iStock.)

Who Are You Teaching To?

Once you have the foundation of where you want to go, consider your audience. Approximately how many students do you have? Do you know their background? Have they been through formal education or were they home-schooled? Do any have prior college experience? Will you have a chance to meet them personally, perhaps at an orientation or in another class? Knowing your students up front before class can offer tremendous guidance and decrease the guessing game when creating various activities. For example, if you have a class of nursing students, and know that most of them have been an MA, a CNA, or a paramedic, how you begin your approach will differ from if you have a group straight out of high school with no prior medical experience. Also, students who have been through formal education have typically been in a classroom where they sit quietly, raise their hands, and ask questions. If you plan on using other approaches, you will need to teach these students how to behave in a nontraditional classroom.

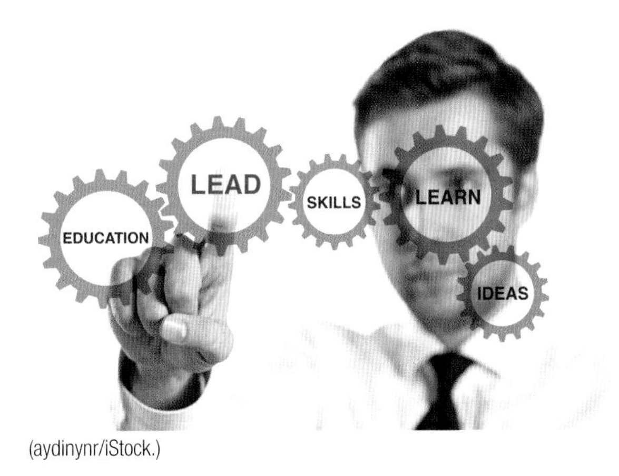

(aydinynr/iStock.)

You will need to prepare for *how* your students learn. As we reviewed in Chapter 1, students learn a variety of ways. In fact, some may have learning challenges, some may excel, some may know their learning style, most may not. In reference to Chapter 1 on learning theories, remember the review of Gardner's theory on multiple intelligences. You learned ways to teach to each of the nine intelligences/learning styles for your various courses. Now is the time to expand on that idea.

Active Learning Versus Passive Learning

You need to know what students already know so you will know what they don't know. An easy format to assess this is by alternating teaching and learning: "you teach me, I teach you, you teach me, I finish teaching you." In this example, the instructor assesses a student's prior learning (you teach me what you know), fills in what they don't recall (I teach you), allows them to show what they *do* know (you teach me), and closes the gap at the end (I finish teaching you). There is no need to teach them information they are already equipped with, but it never hurts to review material to ensure everyone is at the same starting place. By assessing their prior learning, you will be able to adjust your lecture to ensure you cover appropriate material. Offering an initial pop quiz or using small groups to perform a short evaluation of prior learning is an easy way to start off your course and get to know your audience. Having this awareness of what your students already know, you can begin to fill in details and add content in areas they do not know but need to learn. This is where your expertise comes into play; providing short lectures, PowerPoints or videos, and expanding their base knowledge, on the first day gets everyone off to a good start.

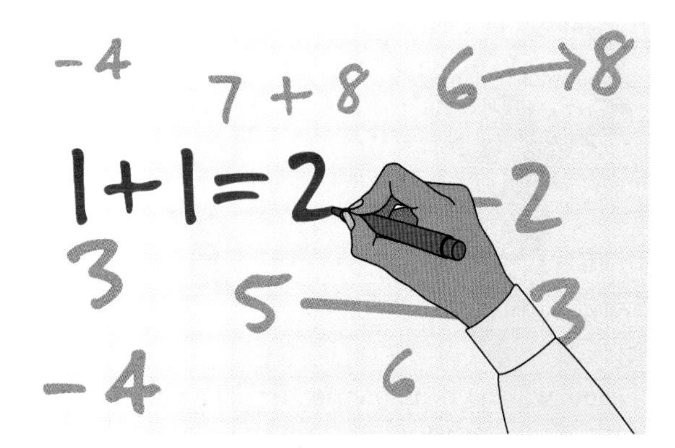

Let's use a math class as an example. If you are teaching medical math, you need to know the comfort level students have with the basics. Presumably everyone will at least be proficient in adding and subtracting, division, and multiplication (regardless of what method they use). However, students may be a bit rusty on portions and percentages and need a review. You may start off with a simple quiz, determine where deficiencies are, then solve a few problems on the whiteboard, reminding students how to calculate percentages from fractions. Perhaps you will then have a few students go to the whiteboard to do some additional problems and offer one more quiz. You will complete this class by reviewing the answers, ensuring students know the steps in solving these math problems. Those who don't might need more one-to-one remediation, not uncharacteristic of your own course.

As we focus on active learning versus passive learning it is important to realize that as much as you are planning your course, you are planning how the students will be engaged. Approximately 20% to 30% of the time you will be lecturing or directing their learning; the remaining 70% to 80% of the time should be directed by the students. This does not mean it's time for you to go to Starbucks; you are still an integral part of the process, and in fact, will have a greater part in the outcome. By carefully planning your course, you will know when you need to step in, when you need to bring students in more, and when you need to get help from outside sources.

Inspiration to Teach

In Chapter 1 you reflected on how you were inspired to teach. Although someone may have nudged you, has anyone shown you effective teaching? Did you have a robust professor who demonstrated great teaching styles? While this may be true, more often new faculty are left with trying to figure out what makes a "good" (effective) teacher. There are a few ways to gain a glimpse of how to be an effective teacher; some are a bit unconventional and others are more obvious. Remember, being an effective teacher doesn't always mean you are the most popular; often it is not until students look back on their education (perhaps even after graduation) that they realize how effective their teacher was. It is then that they appreciate the rigor they went through and are be able to thank you.

An obvious way to demonstrate effective teaching is to be the student—watching other teachers. While your institution may have observation as part of your orientation, it can be helpful if you can attend other lectures or can do so on your own time. If possible, dress up like a student and go to other classes or other colleges (ask the professor if you can sit and observe for a few hours or a day). Sit and listen with a discerning but open mind; be sure it is a subject matter that you are interested in and not necessarily one that you will teach. Infiltrating the classroom as a student gives you the viewpoint of the students, not as a faculty member. This is important as you are looking with the same objectivity and potential for boredom that your students will have. Take copious notes—what did you like, what didn't you like and why. If it were your class, what would you do differently? What effect do you think this different approach would have on the outcome?

While observing an actual class is helpful, sometimes it is nice to look at a perfect world. We have Hollywood to thank for that, as there are various movies that are both inspiring and uplifting. While some are based on actual teachers, others are for sheer enjoyment. Consider watching a movie on powerful teachers, or even transformational coaches. It doesn't have to feel like work but can be funny and encouraging and possibly give you some ideas on how to be unique in your approach. While there are many movies spanning the early 1960s and beyond, a few highlighted ones include *Freedom Writers*, *Sister Act 2*, *Dead Poets Society*, *School of Life*, and *Akeelah and the Bee*; coaching movies include *Coach Carter*, *Remember the Titans*, and *We Are Marshall*. Some of these are based on actual teachers, some are fiction, all have some humor (a necessity for teaching), and hopefully one will help inspire you to think outside the box.

A Variety of Teaching Styles

When considering your teaching style preference, you may need additional resources to help round out your course. If you are a novice teacher, you may not know exactly what style is best for you. Based on your audience, your preferred teaching style may not be the most effective; thus you may have to augment or alter your style. While we will go further into student engagement in Chapter 4, we can begin to incorporate ideas on teaching styles now.

LECTURE

By far the most common teaching style is lecturing. However, even lecturing can be done in a variety of ways. Most lecturers will be situated at the front of the classroom, with either a whiteboard or chalkboard (or some variance), as well as a computer, projector, speakers, and possibly additional technical equipment. Some lectures will be to a very large audience or online and may require a headset or microphone; some may be to a very small class, whereby you will be sitting with your students. Regardless of the setup, the dynamics of the lecture is most important. Be sure to get up and walk around the class or sit at the back of the room for some portion of the class. Immersing yourself in the room with your students can keep their attention for longer and even keep them more interactive. It is important to realize that lectures need to be less than an hour, complete with breaks and other activities. As most people can only listen for a short time, keep in mind your lecture needs to be broken up into other segments so it will be easier for your students to follow along.

Get out of your way when lecturing. Many times, a faculty member drones on about a subject matter, filled with personal anecdotes on how they were involved, and absolutely lose most of the class. If you were an emergency room (ER) nurse, for example, and want to share how crazy the night shift was when you worked there 20 years ago, keep in mind how it would relate to your subject matter. While you may indeed have a great deal of experience in the ER and want to share some gruesome tales or nail-biting experiences, keep the information short and pertinent to the actual topic. You may want to share that the ER is a place to consider if you like a fast-paced environment, where there is constant change and a lot of players involved. For those who appreciate a calmer more organized unit, they may want to consider working at a clinic or even an urgent care facility. If students are keenly interested in your stories, you may elaborate after class or during a break instead of taking valuable class time.

POWERPOINT

As the adage goes, there is imminent death by PowerPoint. However, Microsoft's PowerPoint (PPT) can be a great tool to display slides, images, or be an organized method of presenting facts. However, there are a few rules when using PPT:

- use the slides to only reveal main ideas or statistics,
- use bullet points instead of full sentences,
- ensure there are images or creative artwork to make the slides more interesting,

- use animations, transitions, and music/sounds to keep students' interest,
- keep slides to a small number (based on the time you have),
- keep additional notes hidden so only the faculty member can view for prompting.

Another good rule when using PPT is to allow time for the students to read the slide. Never read the slide or have a student read the slide as this suggests students cannot read on their own (usually not the case when in a college setting). Also, it is helpful to use a pointer and a wireless device to advance the slides, so that no one, especially you, are tethered to the space bar to advance the slides. This also allows you to walk around the room and ensure students are listening (more about this technique in Chapter 4).

If you choose to use PPTs and want to print the slides out, make this an engagement activity. Put two to four slides on a page (to reduce waste) and allow room for students to write in answers. Prompt them during a slide to extrapolate further on the fact or idea—this creates a more active learning experience as the student must pay attention and follow along, and is reminded of this important fact or idea when they are filling in missing information or answer a question. For example, if you are lecturing on community health or sexual reproduction and want to share current facts and statistics on sexually transmitted diseases (STDs), provide a slide with bullet points on these facts but leave room for students to look up gender, age, or geographical location of the highest incidents.

While PPT is a great tool and may come with some of your textbooks, there are other presentation materials that can be used such as Prezi or Keynote. Whichever software program you choose, you need to be very comfortable with how to create the slides or presenting material, as well as how to execute it. Nothing is as embarrassing as having a great presentation, but no familiarity in presenting it. Do not rely on or hope that information technology (IT) personnel will be available, or that your students will be able to assist (even more embarrassing). Using the excuse that you have technical difficulties will lose some respect and credibility; such hiccups could also lose a student's interest, never to be regained. Be sure that you know how to operate the computer and the software program, that you have permission to use it (especially if you use Mac and your institution is Windows based), and that it all works together; make time to practice days before your class to prevent any further frustrations.

HANDS ON

Depending upon the subject matter of your course, consider including a few hands-on activities, demonstrations, or skills that students can do. It can be as easy as using building blocks, actual equipment, or other means to extrapolate what you are lecturing on; you must be clear on what they will use the item for. Take again the math class we spoke of; perhaps you have measuring cups or bring in brownies or a pie to review portions and fractions. Students would be able to use this hands-on activity to realize that 0.5 = 50% = half of a cup, or that a brownie/pie can be divided into fourths, eighths, or whatever measurement you want (not to mention students love to eat!). This gives students a real-world example of an abstract idea and allows them to begin to connect the pieces cognitively (both literally and figuratively).

VIDEOS

With the ease of using YouTube and other online videos, faculty have access to a myriad of already recorded demonstrations and teaching snippets. Even if you were to lecture on the same topic in the same way, including these short videos often reinforces what you are lecturing on and can add value as well as validation to your lecture. When considering any video, it is important to review it prior to using it. Be sure that it is accessible via your institution's computer, that it is free (there are many topics out there), and that you have it cued up outside of any commercials. Also check the video to determine if there is an endorsement included in it—several large companies will have free and enlightening videos on a topic, but with a skewed perspective. Your video needs to remain objective unless you are using it to demonstrate a particular viewpoint; if so, you should likewise show the opposite side for balance. This is especially useful when discussing an emotionally charged topic, such as euthanasia, abortion, or homelessness. Students should never be swayed to only see one side of an issue. As the facilitator, it is your responsibility to bring about a wider perspective for your students.

While short videos can be engaging and are appropriate, careful consideration should be made before using movies. While there are many great movies, including documentaries that can support your material, they are often lengthy and can take up much of your class time. As tempting as this might be, it is not a good practice. Some students will actually oppose watching movies during class time, as they "can do this at home"; other students, especially those who work, may even fall asleep during the movie. Without any activities associated with watching, movies are a passive form of learning (if indeed learning is taking place). Instead of watching the entire movie during class, consider assigning this activity as homework. Provide questions to guide the learner while they are watching, or start the movie off in class, assigning the rest for homework, and resuming the review the next day (complete with the Q&A). A good example of this exercise is for a developmental class in biology or psychology. The movie, *The Curious Case of Benjamin Button*, provides a unique story that has many topics which could be included in either or both classes. However, this movie is over 2.5 hours long—far too long to be included in a class. A better idea is for the instructor to start the movie with some simple guidance, allow students to watch it at home with their Q&A handout, and resume the discussion on another class day. You would want to ensure that all students have access to a TV or computer and can download a movie for free (never assume this). You may also be able to offer free watching at the campus (after class) if your institution allows it.

While using movies during class time may not be wise, having students make movies is certainly fair game. There are various apps and software programs they can use to create mini-movies, infomercials, and short videos. These activities also foster critical thinking, active learning, and allow students to insert their own creativity into their learning. When assigning a movie or infomercial for students to make, be sure to include a clear set of rules and expectations. There should never be profanity, nudity, or anything illegal or offensive, regardless of what the subject matter is. Check with your institution to determine if any waivers must be signed if other people are being filmed, especially the vulnerable population (e.g., children or the elderly). You will also need to create a rubric that clearly delineates the point structure for this activity (we will discuss this further in Chapter 7).

OUTSIDE SPEAKERS

While you are probably an excellent orator, even you can get tired of your own voice. No one says *you* must do all the talking—consider your community. There are many resources that offer guest speakers at no charge. Many of these feel they want to give back and see emerging college students as fertile ground in which to do so. What better way to impart knowledge that you must disseminate to the community and the next generation than by simply being invited into a classroom. Check your local service agencies such as the Rotary Club, Teamsters, and your local Veteran's agency. Many of these offer speakers on a wide range of topics from folks who have been in the industry. Not only will students gain additional knowledge, the speaker will also feel validated that they were able to help others. Think outside the box—explore other resources that may be more unconventional but would make an impact on your student's learning. Consider a class about cardiac health, or death and dying; you may want to invite hospice or grievance counselors; you may also want to invite therapy comfort dogs or schedule a field trip to a funeral home to provide the bigger picture of how people cope with death. These are the makings of an instructor who ties in what they have to say to what they want students to learn.

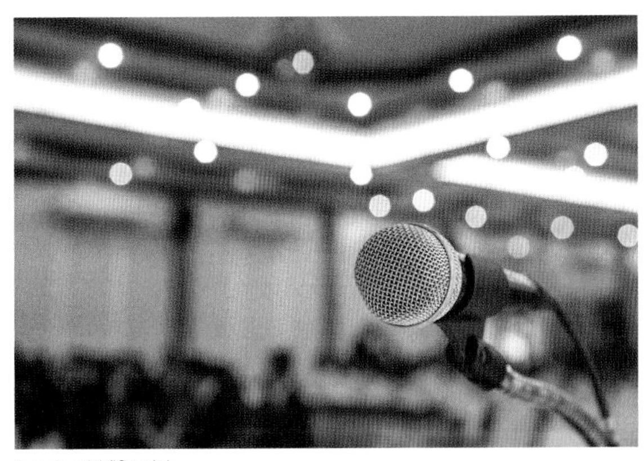

(smolaw11/iStock.)

Other free resources for guest speakers can be found online. TED Talks is one of the more commonly used online resources available for all faculty; while their focus was originally on topics that included technology, entertainment, and design (thus the acronym), TED has expanded to include a variety of speeches on science, current events, and other topics that pertain to the college student. These talks are often short (less than 30 minutes) and should be reviewed just like the videos previously mentioned. Note: TED is responsible for the review of the content submission and may choose to remove a talk from its library. If you are using a particular talk, always check to ensure it is still part of their library before assuming it is.

SMALL GROUPS

Your lectures will be better understood if you pause and allow time for students to process the information. This can easily be done with small informal groups. For example, after reviewing an especially intense subject, ask your students to sit together in groups of two to three (no more than five) and review what they just learned. Have one person be the moderator, one the scribe, and one be ready to share with the larger class. Provide them with three to four specific questions to reflect on and to share within their small group, and then have them share with the larger class. The questions could be something like: What do you feel is the most important aspect of this topic? What do you think you know after hearing this lecture? What do you still want to know? You may not have time for all the groups to share, but at least allow a significant portion of the class to share so that the students realize there was a purpose to the exercise. Write (or have a student write) the summation of all groups' sharing on the whiteboard so they can see how similar their answers are. This may even stimulate additional discussions or provide guidance for the faculty to clarify students' learning or ensure you cover what they still want to know.

GAMES AND PUZZLES

While it may seem unconventional, research has shown that when adults are having fun (just like children) they are learning and are able to retain the information better. This notion is not only hard for some faculty to grasp, but also for some students (you mean I can have fun in the classroom?). There are a variety of games and puzzles available online, as well as using simple everyday items like blocks, balloons, board games, and actual puzzles. Consider a class on communication or professionalism: have small groups of students put together a children's jigsaw puzzle of 100 pieces or less without speaking; allow them a designated time to complete this task. To make it more challenging, remove the box so they cannot see the final picture of the puzzle. This activity requires little preparation and but can launch a variety of discussions regarding teamwork, how the group started (or completed) the project without words, and how we can intuitively work together. Activities like these often have bragging rights as the best reward, but at least get faculty (and students) thinking outside the box.

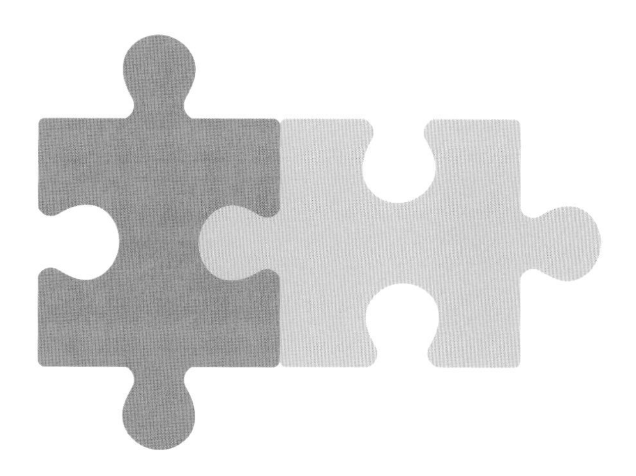

Elsevier has various games and activities available online, based on each textbook; go to your textbook online, under Teacher or Student Resources, and see what the author has listed. If you do not have time to offer this activity or game in class, you can direct students to the Student Resources and assign an activity as homework. Plan ahead and let students know that you will start the next class based on what they learned from this assignment and use it to jump start your next class. Students often enjoy these activities, but also need to know there is a purpose or point attached. Knowing that this will be the first thing you cover the next class day provides a rationale for completing the homework.

CRITICAL THINKING EXERCISES

Similar to games and puzzles requiring you to think outside the box, critical thinking exercises will require that students look at things from a different perspective. These activities can be embedded in your lecture, as a side activity in individual formats, or be team focused. They can be used separately, much like games and puzzles, or parallel the subject you are teaching. Chapter 5 will go into more detail about the rationale for these activities, as well as some exercises to consider. For now, be sure to include these in your course frequently to promote the higher order of thinking you desire.

CASE STUDIES

No matter what subject you are teaching, there are plenty of case studies that support your topic. You can use already created ones, edit them, or create your own based on the topics you are covering. You can also have other students create them, either from the same class (but a different group) or from a different class, alumni, or even a different campus. The idea is to have students apply what they are learning to real world examples, use their critical thinking skills (hence the need to sharpen those skills), and acquire a greater understanding of the material.

Case studies will work more effectively with some classes than others. Consider the class whereby you have both nontraditional and traditional students; grouping them in a variety of small groups to review the study can bring forth their individual talents, strengths, and experience. In reviewing the case, their personal perception, based on their generation, can offer different outcomes on how they will handle the case, or at least provide a lively discussion for the group members.

DEBATES

Though not all classes will support opposing viewpoints, those that have the time and subject matter can benefit from students forming teams and debating an issue. As discussed in the videos section, topics that have opposing viewpoints such as euthanasia and abortion provide alternate perspectives that draw from a variety of angles including culture, religion, family dynamics, and upbringing, as well as modern health care. In a debate there is an affirmative (the side that agrees with the issue) and the negative, or opposing side, that disagrees with the issue. There are actual rules when debating, such as: students must research current trends and withhold opinions, they must speak professionally and not shout at one another, and they cannot refer to the opposing side as being wrong—that is the whole premise to the debate. No side is right or wrong.

In addition to the teams supporting each "side," there should be a moderator and an audience. Consider, for example, if you held a debate on the topic of the right to die. While each team may have their own personal opinion, they must use current laws, medical knowledge, and a focused situation on when a person has the choice (or not) to request assistance in dying. As you can probably imagine, while this requires little preparation on the instructor's side, it requires very clear direction for the students to know their boundaries. For example, in this hypothetical debate, the circumstances must first be clearly outlined as there are many situations in which no one would agree that a person has a choice to end their life (committing suicide). Children, the mentally ill, or other populations may be excluded from the argument. The faculty must allow a great deal of guidance, allow time, and offer oversight as the teams perform their research. Notwithstanding, the students in the audience likewise have to do their own research so they can accept that the opposing teams are accurate in their presentation and also glean enough understanding so that they can ask pertinent questions. Obviously, the class has to be long enough for you and your students to have ample time to perform this debate; however, many courses can accommodate this, including online courses, if the faculty is well prepared.

INDEPENDENT STUDY

While you will be directing the overall learning, there is something to be said for students conducting additional learning within the context of what they want to learn. Not all students will be able to perform independent study effectively, especially in a face-to-face classroom. Independent study requires a little more discipline and a yearning to learn more than the prescribed material. You can certainly create such a desire for students to learn more and offer additional learning opportunities. However, it is often helpful to allow this to be an optional assignment. On the contrary, online learning often requires a great deal of independent study and is more conducive to this form of learning as students have a less restrictive environment. Independent study is often used when there is a great deal of research or literature review needed or a topic has so much to offer that it simply cannot be reviewed in its entirety during your course. Providing guides for further research or offering probing questions will facilitate independent study and guide the eager learner without overwhelming them.

FIELD TRIPS

Depending upon where you live and the subject matter, consider scheduling a field trip to a local business or museum that supports your topic. These resources are often hidden jewels and are usually found by doing some digging (all puns intended) via community centers and local agencies. Medical museums, pharmacy museums, math museums, and even zoos can readily provide interesting and engaging activities that complement your course material. Be sure to call ahead to determine hours, prices, and whether a docent or tour guide is available. Some facilities will have additional resources if they know you are an educator, so be clear on what you are there for. Most facilities will offer group discounts or special pricing (including free admission) if they are scheduled in advance; offer to go during off-peak times to optimize the students' learning experience (it's much more fun when you don't have to battle a large crowd). Once again, be sure you are clear on what your institution will pay for and their policies on reimbursement for students. A good rule of thumb is that students shouldn't have to pay large amounts, especially if they are already paying for this course. Based on your school's policy you may be able to hold a bake sale or rummage sale to raise funds, so no one is out of pocket. Community members are more supportive of these special fundraising events when they are aware of what the cause is. Another option is to consider having a local business sponsor your class; again, check your school's policy to ensure you are compliant.

Chicken Soup for the Teacher

All of these strategies can be used at a certain time during your course; however, planning is the most important strategy. As faculty, you are the one guiding the learning and must see the direction your course is taking. This also means you must take care of yourself. As simple as it sounds, faculty can spend a large amount of time exploring the earlier resources, calling and emailing contacts, and usually do this during their free time. While it may not be realistic to do this research only during office hours, be judicious in your quest and time invested. Confer with fellow faculty to determine what or whom have they used; do they have some contacts they have already used that might be appropriate? What are some outside resources that have already helped your department? Are any of them experts that can also serve as a guest speaker?

Regardless of how excited you are to begin your teaching career it is important that you are prudent in your planning, as you can easily overextend yourself. Self-care is essential to ensure your enthusiasm is balanced with reality. The newly hired faculty member who has planned a 20-hour course for a 2-hour class and has devoted their entire weekend on rolling it out Monday morning may become quickly deflated when students come in and are barely awake, much less enthused about doing a bunch of games or listening to yet another speaker. Don't take it personally; don't get into the "shoulda, coulda, woulda's," and most importantly, don't give up. Although it should go without saying, be sure that you practice what you preach: get plenty of rest, exercise, and emotional support as you begin your teaching journey. You will need an objective sounding board as you try out various teaching techniques and find your niche. Remember, never take it personally if your class does not learn, enjoy, or revel in the day you planned. Brush it off and plan better for the next day. As a human, you are entitled to have an off day too; learn from this experience and grow from it. You will be a better teacher because of it.

What Do You Want to Teach?

What do *you* want students to do in this course?

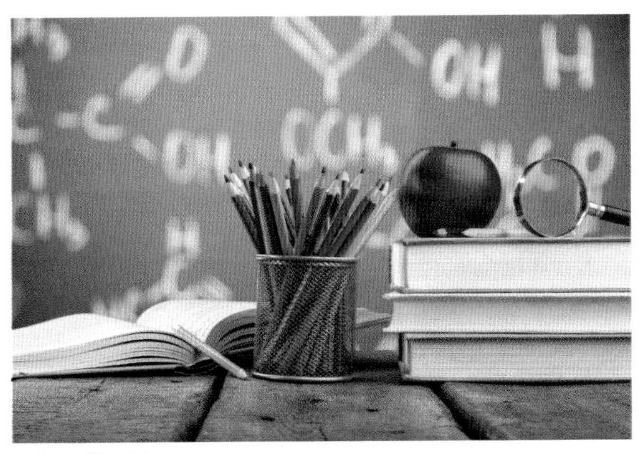

(artisteer/iStock.)

While we must adhere to formal goals and objectives, each class will also include your personal desire for the students. It could be that you want them to work on their teambuilding, self-confidence, time management, or professionalism. It could be that you want them to have fun, especially on the first day of class, a class right after a midterm, or at the end of each class. Maybe you want them to lead several of the classes and instill great leadership qualities. Whatever it is, be sure to align these internal goals with the overall goals for the course. As Stephen Covey says, "begin with the end in mind."

Consider the earlier strategies listed; decide which ones are appropriate for your class, which ones may be a stretch, which ones you do not like (yes, you have permission to not enjoy an activity), and which ones may not be the right fit for this course. You may not be able to use some resources this time but can start creating a resource binder for next time. For example, if you are teaching this class during the winter months and have inclement weather, you may have to wait until springtime to do an outside field trip. Your guest speakers and other resources may not be available at the time you want; while you may have some flexibility with the course, you will want to ensure the guest speaker is as close to the scheduled day you are presenting the topic as possible. It is not prudent to have a guest speaker come 2 to 3 days after the topic as you will have surely brought in new information, thus confusing the students. Because there may be circumstances which are out of your control, it is helpful to begin calendaring your top items that you want. If you are stuck with not acquiring them, you will also learn how far in advance you will have to plan the next time you teach this course.

Your course offers a chance for you to influence your students in a variety of ways. As a result of your course, students will be able to do several things—primarily those listed in the syllabus, IP or LP, in addition to the personal goals you have set for them. How will you bring them to perform the tasks necessary to achieve these goals? How will you know whether or not they have reached these goals? While Chapter 7 will go into assessments, along the way there are tools you can use to ensure you are on course. One of the most obvious and easiest is to simply spend time with your students. Including office hours, be present before and after class, and occasionally have a brown bag day, which will allow you to be more approachable to your students. This can also elicit casual conversations surrounding the course, how students are learning, and any suggestions they may have. While this is entirely optional, it is also cautioned that you do not spend a great deal of time outside of class with only certain students. Be available to all students during designated times and ensure these casual conversations are limited; you do not want to set the precedent that you are a buddy or that you have any favorites.

Timing for Your Class

Timing is everything—and this is true in a classroom. You cannot simply walk into a class, purge your brain and reveal all there is to know about a subject, expect students to pay attention, be interested, and recall all of that information. There is a great deal more finesse involved, as you must understand the whole human being who is trying to learn. Chances are they have a family or at least a social circle outside of class, they may have jobs or other commitments, and have other things to do than attend class. Even if they don't, they can think of a hundred things to do other than sit and listen to you. So why should they listen to you? Yes, they probably need your class to obtain their degree or certificate, but that is not enough to keep them interested, motivated, or committed to listening. You, as the facilitator of their learning, must make it interesting, challenging, and meet some expectations. In private colleges, especially, students feel they have paid a lot of money to get a degree/certificate. What they may not realize is that they paid to get an opportunity to be educated; however, you are the one guiding their education—make it worth their money.

Timing during your class needs to be planned out. While this may seem obvious, you will need to plan your breaks, your non-lecture material, and your downtime activities. In fact, little of your time needs to be about you. This is not to bruise your ego, but to be realistic about how long students can listen to even the most enjoyable lecture. Research has shown that most adults can tolerate less than 20 minutes of lecture without roaming into internal and external distractions. That's a very short attention span, probably due to our immediate cyberworld. Think about it: if you have to wait more than 2 minutes for your computer to boot up, it is slow; pizza is delivered within 30 minutes; Amazon Prime delivers almost whatever you want within 2 days, and even retailers are offering free delivery. Everything revolves around how fast things are—this is the world in which we now live. Education has to be equally as responsive, because our economy and its patrons have become used to this "immediacy." This is not to advocate avoiding exercises that take time, such as journaling and self-reflection; just as you are doing as part of this program, you can savor those moments and allow the ideas and thoughts to bubble up naturally. Even so, there should be a time limit to prevent you from getting too far off track or wandering in your inner thoughts.

In Preparation for Class

As you are planning your course, you need to follow a few simple rules of behavior yourself. Some of these might be formally addressed in your institution's policy or faculty handbook, but we are listing the important ones just in case.

1. Be on time—that means at least 30 minutes early. Ensure you are there ahead of the start of class time for your students, in case they have questions or need clarification.
2. Have all of your handouts, printouts, forms, games, notes, PPTs, etc. ready. Don't be running back and forth printing or copying. Even if you were early but still needed to keep running back and forth means you were unprepared.
3. Check the computers, screens, and any other technology before you start class—everyday. Overnight there may have been an update or a reset and what worked yesterday may not work today. Don't brush it off as technical difficulties—be ready ahead of time and let IT know if indeed there are technical difficulties.
4. Gather all of your materials before starting class: pens, whiteboard markers, erasers, laser pointers, anything you need for the class. Don't keeping going back and forth to fetch more—bring it all initially.
5. Have a roster and/or seating arrangement ahead of time. Know who is expected to be there and assign seating if necessary. If there is not assigned seating, consider having a name plate in front of each student so you know their names.
6. Teach at a good pace, with good dialect. The best way to determine this is to simply ask your students: Does that make sense? Am I going too fast? Do you need me to repeat that? This is especially true if you have a different dialect or accent—can they understand you? A faculty member from New York can struggle with a class in Alabama just as much as someone from Japan can struggle with a class in India. Our melting pot of global communication is wonderful but can present some challenges.

7. If you choose to use a presentation software like PPT, adhere to the points mentioned earlier. Be sure to have the packet of printed slides (if you choose to do this) along with other materials.
8. Don't have stacks of handouts for students. While they may think that you care and have such a plethora of knowledge waiting for them, unless they use it, they will often toss it in the trash, leave it behind, or allow the dog to eat it. Students can feel very overwhelmed and under-educated with too much information.
9. Don't fake it—students will know if you did not plan! Be organized—that is often the number one complaint from students: their faculty were not prepared. If a student feels they can stay at home and learn the same thing on their own, why should they come to class?
10. Dress professionally—you probably have to adhere to your college/institutions' dress code; take it to the next level. While comfort is important, don't look like a student. You shouldn't try to fit in with their style, clearly you have your own (regardless of what era it is from). On the flip side, leave the three-piece suit for weddings and funerals—you don't need to look like you are making a statement either. You also want to be comfortable, as you will most likely be on your feet for hours. You want to be professional; your first impression to your students will speak loud and clear. How you dress can also influence your students; while they may have a lenient dress code compared to yours, you can instill a sense of pride in how they outwardly appear to others.

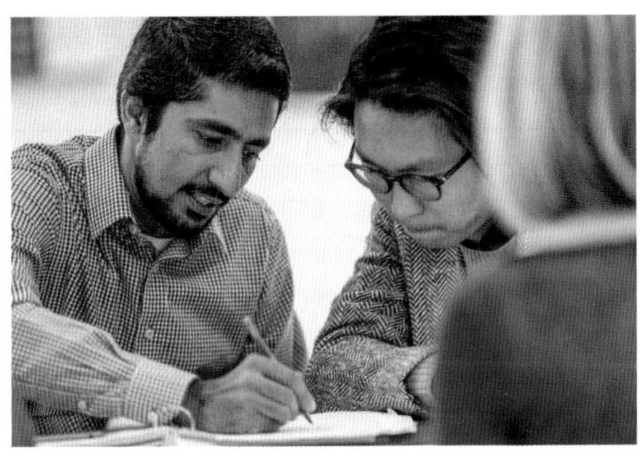
(FatCamera/iStock.)

Plan every day—yes, *every* day. You may find that some days go according to plan and others fall short. By having an overall plan each day, you can accommodate each differential from the previous day and ensure there is continuity. You will also get a sense of the pace your class needs—perhaps you are going too slow or too fast, perhaps they have more questions and need a time period to review the answers. Whatever the tempo is, adjust accordingly and move forward, realizing you will need to adjust again once your students become in tune with your teaching style. As stated previously—absolutely do not take it personally or feel that you have failed if you must make these adjustments. This is actually good feedback as it will continue to guide you in future planning. It is better to over-plan than under-deliver.

What If?

There is a saying, "in every world there is a disconnect between the real and the ideal." Your first day may be a flop; you may run out of all 20 hours of activities in the first 4 hours; you may find that no activity is well received by your students. Your days may be full of the greatest fears of "what if's?" Don't let this deter you or allow you to derail. It happens, even to the most prepared instructor, the seasoned faculty, and the most knowledgeable. The one thing to remember is that you are the teacher, and you are still responsible for the course. So what if you have to punt and redirect students; who cares if you don't get to the eight packets of handouts you copied and stapled at midnight last night (another reason not to have so many stacks of handouts!), will anyone know what you didn't get to do in class other than you? And if they knew, would it matter?

All faculty get frustrated from time to time; they may fall short of their plans and may even have to chart another path in their course. What prevails, and what your students will notice, is your attitude about it. If you are angry, disappointed, discouraged, or even confused, your students will sense your negative energy. This negativity can deflate their enthusiasm and may become an obstacle to their learning. It is important to remain positive, perhaps even have a sense of humor about it (if appropriate). Consider, for example, an instructor who realizes a particular learning exercise is going awry. Instead of getting flustered, the instructor ditches the prescribed lesson and jokingly admits "Well, this wasn't what I planned for you today." The instructor tells the class it is time to regroup and asks if anyone has a better idea than that? Students may have more respect for the honesty and willingness to persevere even though things didn't go as planned. If your ego isn't tied up in the planning, and you can be open minded, you may even find some really creative ideas from your students. If not, or if you don't like their ideas, always have more in your "toolbox." Based on these ideas, it's time we stock your toolbox for planning.

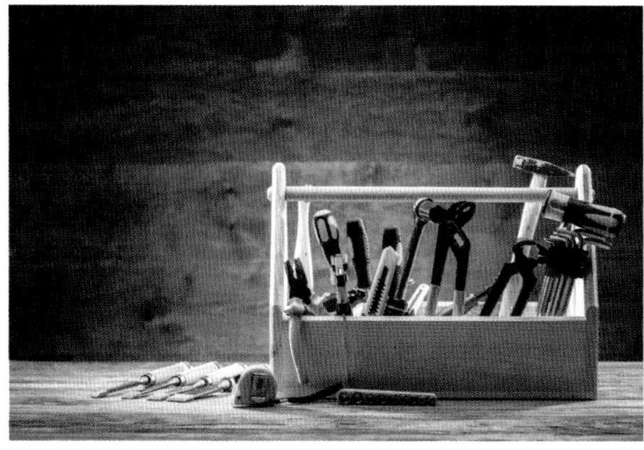

(AndreyPopov/iStock.)

Journal—Self-reflection

1 *Stocking your toolbox*

a. In planning your course there are certain things you need to have ready to use or may need to learn how to use. Regardless of whether you are a novice or more experienced teacher, you have an arsenal already in your toolbox. Write down the ones that you can use to guide your next course:

____

____

____

____

____

____

____

____

____

____

____

____

b. What additional items do you feel you need to add to your toolbox? These can be internal things such as time management, prioritization, and other professional or social skills.

____

____

____

____

2 *IP, LP, and syllabus*

We covered items you have to include in your teaching, such as the IP, LP, and the syllabus. Take a moment to review these in tandem with one another. You will need to ask someone from your institution to assist you with these, as it is imperative you have the most current plans to compare.

The name of your course:______________________________

a. What are some discrepancies you see between the IP, LP, and your syllabus?

b. Realizing that you may or may not have had input for your syllabus, does it read well? If possible, have a non-student look at it and tell you how they read the expectations, assignments, and plan. Does it make sense to them?

c. Are you clear on what is on the tests and quizzes and the expectations for the assignments and any other activities? What questions do you have about the answers, the grading policy or rubric, or how to score the assignment?

Knowing the expectations, how to grade, and where to find answers puts an added tool of knowledge in your toolbox!

3 *Your audience*

Have you had a chance to investigate who your students are? Have you met them? Write down the characteristics you are aware of, such as age range, culture, background, and gender. There is no need to be exact, but it can be helpful information to guide you. Teaching STDs to a group of 50- to 70-year-old retired men is a lot different from teaching the same subject to a mixed group of Catholic females aged 18 to 22 years.

4 *Your observations*

a. When you observed the class as a student, what did you notice that you liked? What did you notice that you didn't like or that was a turnoff? What were some teaching styles that you want to add to your toolbox?

b. Considering the above class, what would you definitely have done differently if this were your class?

5 *Teaching styles*

We have reviewed a variety of teaching styles, methods, and practices. While you may use some, you may defer others to another class. Regardless of the class you are teaching right now, consider each of the following and write down when you might include this style, and what specific resources you would use. Investing the time to put the detail in this exercise now will add many tools to your box, ones that you may use in the inevitable "What if's" or may find as a welcome gift to yourself down the road.

a. Lecture: how will you lecture? What steps will you take to ensure your lecture is able to capture the attention of your students? What tools do you need to ensure your lecture is on task?

____

____

____

____

____

b. PPT: are you using a PPT or other presentation? How many slides? Have you reviewed this PPT or recently created it?

____

____

____

____

____

c. Video/Movies: which movies or videos are appropriate for your class? Are your students able to create their own mini-movie or infomercial? Use this space to write all of the video/movies that might be pertinent. Include where to obtain movies, such as Netflix, Amazon, and Hulu. Be very specific about YouTube videos, as they often have similar titles.

____

____

____

____

____

____

____

____

____

d. Speakers/TED talks: have you thought about outside speakers? Which ones would you use? What classes would they be best suited for? List the resources and their contact information below.

____

____

____

____

____

What TED talks are appropriate for your classes? List the course, the TED talk title, and the TED talk author beside it. For easier future reference, ensure you are very specific in these details as they may help you find the right talk later.

e. Small groups: what are some small group discussions you could use? What class would they be best suited for?

f. Games/puzzles: list at least five games or puzzles that you would be able to use. Include Elsevier's already embedded games based on your textbook; list the game and the author. If using an outside game, list the source and where to find it later for easier reference.

g. Critical thinking exercises: although we will delve into this more in Chapter 5, what ideas do you have now about critical thinking exercises? Do you have some resources that you have used or that you have found that can be used to stimulate critical thinking?

h. Case studies: case studies can be observed, written, or played out. What case studies do you have that can be used for your course? What other case studies might be appropriate for a later course? What other case studies do you want your students to explore?

i. Debates: as previously discussed, debates must have an affirmative side (in agreement) and a negative side. First, consider the topic. Second, what are the opposing sides? Third, what especially would you have your students learn from this exercise?

Topic:

Affirmative:

Negative:

Important details to learn:

j. Independent study: while you are guiding the learning, include some outside activities or other independent learning that can be done. Consider students who are either extremely interested, need more of a challenge, or who might even need remediation on a subject. Where would you send them (the Internet or to library), based on your course?

k. Field trips: what is your institution's policy regarding field trips? What field trips do you have planned? Where would you go? Who is the contact? Does this cost money? If so, how do you plan on raising funds?

6 *TLC for you:*

List at least five things you will to do take care of yourself.

7 *What do you want to teach?*
Despite the things you have to teach, list at least three things you also want students to learn.

8 *What if?*
The most important tool is the one you may rarely pull out but is your go-to activity when all else fails. List at least four activities that are not course specific but could span a variety of courses to build self-esteem, professionalism, or simply have fun.

Regardless of whether this is your first course, or if you have taught several courses, it is important that you feel prepared to teach *this* course. What else do you feel you need in order to be ready? What questions do you still have—whether about the logistics of your class or your teaching style?

Be stubborn about your goals and
flexible about your methods.
Unknown

Chapter 3

Classroom Management

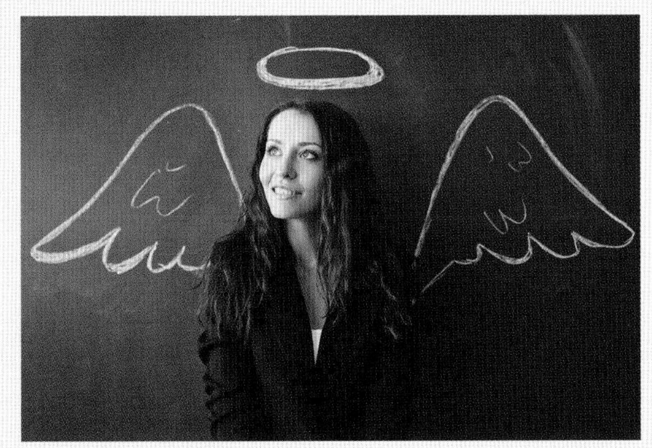

(chesterf/iStock.)

When you think of that perfect classroom, where everyone is sitting in class, eagerly listening and waiting for your lecture, wide eyed and attentive, it's time to check your reality. Despite the hard work you put into your course planning from Chapter 2, the reality is that you may not reach some, any, or all students. Some may have their own agenda, some may not be motivated, and others may simply be fatigued. Before you throw down the book, give up, and get discouraged, let's review some basic points from Chapter 1 about your class.

1. Consider your audience—how do *your* students learn?
2. What motivates your students?
3. Are their basic needs being met? (Hint: remember Maslow's hierarchy of needs.)

If your students are not interested, or are hungry or tired, or feel that the lecture is boring (or all of the above), you will be hard pressed to keep them interested. While we will discuss student engagement in Chapter 4, it is often at this time that faculty see issues creep up regarding classroom management. After all, if everyone were engaged, management of the classroom would be easy—right? Regardless of the activities you have designed, some students simply may not be on board (or at least not yet). Let's identify some of the culprits.

What Is Classroom Management?

Classroom management is the faculty's ability to manage the classroom, primarily the behavior of the students, to ensure the entire classroom environment is conducive to learning for all students. It encompasses both behavior management (the management of each student's behavior) as well as classroom management (managing the entire class so that it is conducive to learning). These two terms, though seemingly intertwined, comprise the crux of overall classroom management. When there is disruption, it can interfere with even the most engaged student's attention. Mismanagement of the classroom can also create legal issues, ethical concerns, and could be grounds for disciplinary action—not just for your students, but for you. It is important that you know how to handle the classroom with respect for all persons, in adherence with your institution's policy, and with a sense of competence. No one wants to be the bad guy, and enforcing rules may not make you teacher of the year; but it is your responsibility to maintain a safe and cordial place for all students to learn. If students begin to question their boundaries, nudge their limits, and behave in an inappropriate manner, it needs to be addressed immediately; otherwise it could be seen as approval and may promote further negative behaviors. Classroom management covers such behaviors as tardiness, absenteeism, talking out of turn or disrespectfully, or simply not doing the work. It also covers legal issues such as drugs or alcohol, bullying, and violence in the classroom. It is important to be clear that you are not considered the classroom policeman, but you are mandated to report any illegal activity.

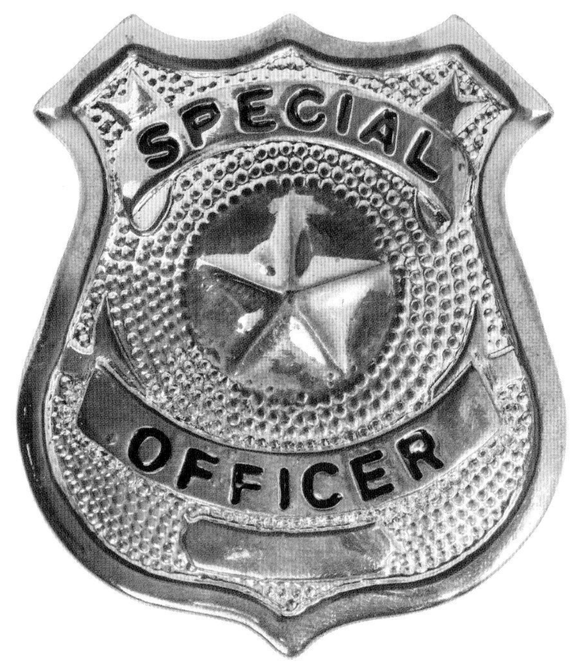

(UroshPetrovic/iStock.)

What Are Your Expectations of Class?

Before we go into managing classroom behavior, think about your expectations of the class. Once again, we must consider how *you* were taught. Was your instructor strict, perhaps even with physical force (a ruler comes to mind)? Did the teacher raise their voice if students weren't paying attention or did students get swatted with that ruler? Were students called out if they were late, fell asleep, or were considered sassy? Did your school have detention after class for those who weren't obeying the rules? These tactics were used from the mid-1900s to primarily the 1980s; however, despite the negative exposure from civil right activists, some school districts continue to employ some form of corporal punishment. It may be surprising to discover that most states can incorporate their own rules and the consequences for not abiding by such rules, including physical forms of punishment. However, it is generally frowned upon as there are more effective measures to promote positive behavior. Nonetheless, your vision of how students should behave, and how they should be reprimanded, must be considered.

While the self-reflection at the end of this chapter allows you to write down expectations, begin to think about how you want your class to look. Do you see them engaging with each other, chatting, smiling, expanding on each other's ideas and having such conversations spark additional interest? Do you see them sitting in small groups, working on various projects, going to the library and coming back with more ideas? Do you see them in the classroom looking to you for answers to their question? Or perhaps, based on the activity, you see all of these as a possibility? What is certain is that you don't see a classroom full of students sleeping on their textbook. While this can be every new teacher's nightmare, it can be prevented, or at least minimized. As mentioned in Chapter 2, careful planning can reduce this opportunity, but will not prevent it from occurring. Knowing how to manage issues that come up during class will ensure your careful planning pays off.

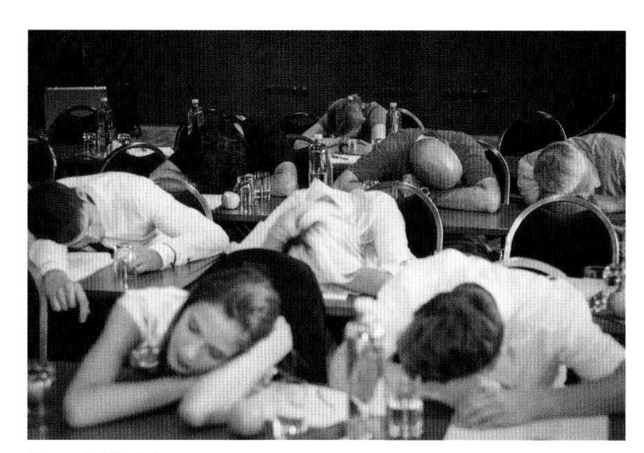

(AzmanL/iStock.)

What Do Your Students Expect?

In addition to your own expectations, consider your audience. What are your students' expectations? Are they in alignment with your expectations? Obviously if they are not congruent, you will have discord. This is not to mean that you will struggle for the duration of your course, but rather, you will need to determine how these expectations can be in better alignment. What were your students told during their admission process? Chances are they met with a variety of people, including financial aid, student services, and an admission representative or a counselor—if so, did those departments share the same expectations you have? Have you taken the time to meet with these departments to compare what is being told to the students? Does your chair or department head feel strongly about discipline, or are they more concerned about facilitating students getting through the course? These conversations need to occur either formally or informally so that you can be sure everyone is telling the students the same thing. Moreover, it is important to review with your students what *their* expectations are—whether it is based on these conversations, preconceived notions of higher education, the institution's reputation, or even what they have heard from their peers.

Some students may have heard your course was an easy class, whereby very little work is expected, and students expect to receive an "A." Being that you are new, other students may have the assumption you don't know how to teach, and thereby will test your stamina. Your school may be struggling with retaining students, and thus some may consider your need to matriculate students more important than their need to behave appropriately and may expect leniency. Some students may have no preconceived notions of you, the school, or the class, but do not feel that they can give 100%; they may have other commitments such as family with young children, jobs, or both. As mentioned in Chapter 2, it is important to ascertain who your audience is, including what they expect of you, the class, and themselves. This should be done before or on the first day of class. You may even have a simple questionnaire that asks these questions:

- What do you expect of me for this class?
- What do you think you will learn as a result of this class?
- What do you expect of yourself during this class?

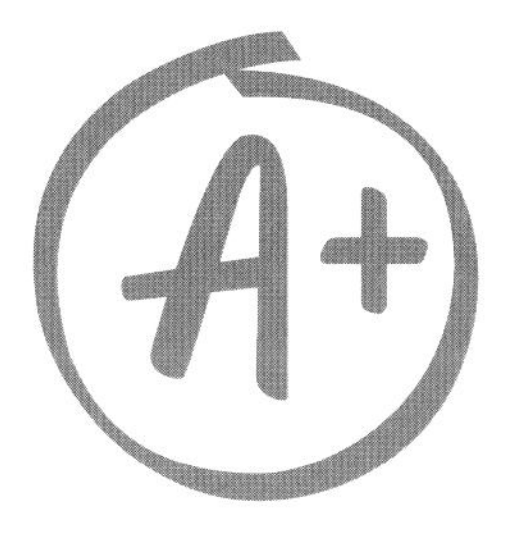

Personal Expectations

There is nothing wrong with having high expectations. It is actually a good thing; however, we need to make sure we can meet such expectation within reason. This includes yourself, your students, and the institution's expectations. If you, your students, and your college all feel the students should pass with an "A" and continue on to the next course, chances are this is not reality. It is expected that some students will excel, some will do a good job, some will do fair, and there may even be students who do not pass. Based on the rigor and content of the material you must cover, the objectives, and what the expectations are of the students, as well as how they are prepared to meet these expectations, will make the difference in whether (or not) they can achieve their goals.

Once you have identified your personal expectation and your students' expectations, consider how realistic they are. Let's take the subject of homework: is it your expectation they read the chapter prior to class and complete all homework assignments? If their expectation is that most of the work is done in class, you will not have your expectations met (neither will the students). Perhaps there is a way to reach a happy medium? Is it possible for you to reduce the homework load? Do you have ample time to allow review of this material in class? If you expect them to review the chapter and can make time during the first hour of class to do this review, it could meet your goals and theirs. Sometimes your class time isn't this flexible, but you will have to judge which is more important and what wiggle room you have.

Your Institution's Expectations

Your institution's expectations are set; often they are nonnegotiable and cover multiple campuses. These expectations, called a code of conduct, are found in the college catalog and are usually very clear, regardless of personal interpretation. For this reason, it is important to verify the intention of the policies set forth, as well as any grievance, contract violation, or dismissal policy. These expectations, as mentioned in Chapter 2, should also be reiterated in your syllabus. It should be absolutely clear, even repetitive, what the conduct and learning expectations are on campus, in the classroom, and between faculty and students. This is true for all learning platforms, even online learning. Online discussions and chat rooms, video conferencing, and even tutorial sessions should not tolerate misconduct by teachers or students. There must be an underlying respect for all people, the environment, and the institution; lack of such respect can disrupt learning.

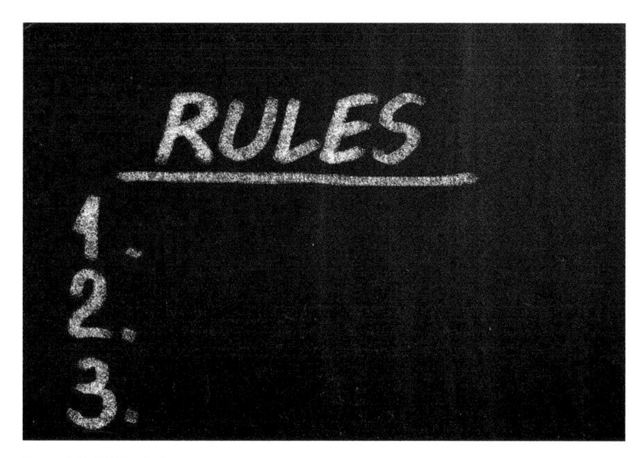

(marrio31/iStock.)

Because there is a constant change in legal wording, diversity, inclusion, student's rights, and the global and governing planet in which we live, most institutions choose to put their catalogs and handbooks online. When reviewing expectations, make sure your students understand this catalog is fluid, meaning that the catalog may be worded one way today, but it may have changed from 3 months ago when they were enrolled, and will probably change again. While these changes are often minor, sometimes a consequence, resource, or other expectation has changed. It is not always clear what changes have been made, but it is important that students (and faculty) realize they are being constantly held to these expectations. You will usually be notified when these changes occur so you can inform your students—for example, if the prior attendance policy changed from students being counted absent if they were more than 30 minutes late, to students now being marked absent if they miss more than 1 hour of lecture, it would be imperative that students realize this discrepancy. Even though another 30 minutes seems minor, it can make a huge difference to a single parent who is struggling trying to get to childcare and doesn't realize being late could cause an absence, versus being marked tardy.

In addition to what you can locate in writing (such as your catalog or handbook), it is important to sit down with your manager to ensure you understand the intentions of the institution. As mentioned, if there is a decline in attendance or in students matriculating, your institution may waiver on enforcing rules, as they feel by doing so they can keep their students. While this often has the opposite effect, you must consider the support you will or will not receive by enforcing your own rules. Most students behave better with more structure, clearer expectations, and consistency when such expectations are enforced. However, those who want to challenge authority will see a loophole if they feel you and your manger or leadership team don't back your play. Never get into a power struggle with students or management or feel that you are the sole disciplinarian. You are their teacher; any tug-of-war with willpower will leave you deflated, frustrated, and could jeopardize your position. Stay focused on what is expected and supported by your leadership team. It will be easier to enforce and allow you to remain more objective.

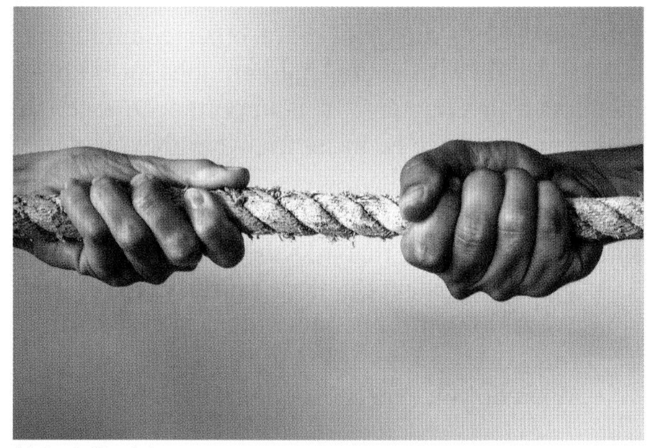
(kieferpix/iStock.)

What You Observe

Hopefully you will have an opportunity to see how your students interact with others, including you or other representatives from the institution. This can help you see who might be a bit shy, or more outgoing, or who seems cheerful and bubbly, and who seems to question everything. It is important to look objectively and not with any judgment; this is a sneak preview of their personalities, not an opportunity to annotate who needs corrective action. In fact, your initial instincts may be off, but you can affirm this later. On the first day of class, or orientation, are there some students who stroll in late, seemingly unaware that this behavior may be disruptive? Or are there some who seem frantic that they are not there on time? These are behaviors that can be addressed one-to-one after letting the entire class know your expectation of attendance including late policies. Do students raise their hands to ask a question or do they shout out their question/answer? Which do you prefer them to do? Do students willingly get up and go to the restroom or step out to use their phone during your lecture? Would you prefer they wait until break time to do so? Be clear, respectful, but honest.

These behaviors, if given the opportunity to observe them prior to class or on the first day, need to be reinforced with your expectations. Often, the instructor may not get a chance to review expectations prior to observing them, so don't hold students accountable until you have had a chance to be clear. For example, if a student comes in late (with or without an apology), don't use that opportunity to say "Gee, now is a good time to go over how I feel about tardiness." This will single out the tardy student and may start your relationship off in a negative fashion; it also labels the student as someone who doesn't obey rules or isn't supportive of you. On the contrary, this may be the only instance whereby the student was late, and the student already feels embarrassed, guilty, and remorseful of their behavior—these feelings are punishments enough to correct the behavior.

What Your Students Observe

When reviewing your expectations, be sure you walk the talk. If you do not tolerate tardiness, be on time; if you despise gossiping, don't start or listen to rumors. As mentioned in Chapter 2, be sure you are prepared in all areas. Whatever you expect of your students, meet them at the next level. If you consider yourself as a role model, your students will have someone to model their behavior after. As a role model or mentor, you are guiding their behavior as much as you are guiding learning. It may very well be that your students do not have a positive role model or someone who acts professionally. Keep in mind they may come from various backgrounds and upbringings; their definition of respect may come from a very different perspective. Often times when students are asked why they behave in an unprofessional manner, they refer to their parents who had no other expectation of them; such behavior went unnoticed, was tolerated, or was perceived as acceptable.

The Disconnect

Expectations among students and faculty need to be congruent; you both are held to the same rules regarding appearance, tardiness, and professionalism. If you don't display this, students will lose respect for you and question why they must adhere to rules. Why should a student bother to come to class on time when the teacher is always 10 minutes late? Just because the catalog or the syllabus says so? After an extended period, students will question why they are in a class where the teacher isn't professional. This can decrease their effort and devalue the class; it also leads to self-deprecation and can reduce self-efficacy, self-esteem, and self-respect.

Modeling Positive Behavior

There are many models of positive behavior for you and your students. Hollywood offers these in various movies (be careful which behaviors you model!), but many of your faculty will have a reputation for upholding rules and emulate this in their classroom. These faculty members are usually known for running a tight ship, being firm but fair, and have a reputation that they worked hard for. Once again, it is not your job to be your students' buddy or friend, neither is it your job to be their parent. For those who may have been a parent or a sibling, how you may treat your children or your siblings is different than how a teacher works with students. Because you and your students are all adults, there needs to be more of a mutual understanding of expectations and accountability.

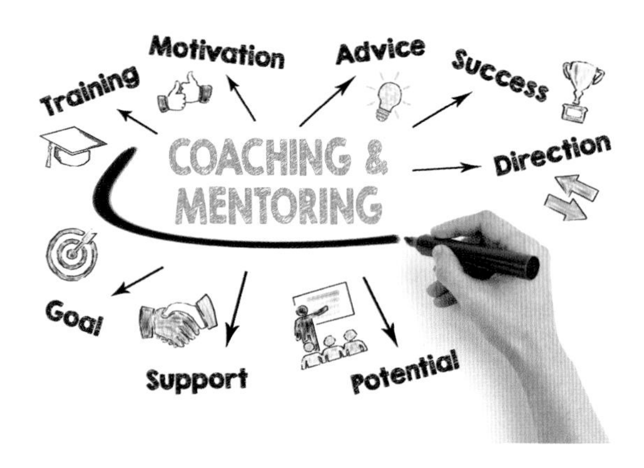

(tumsasedgars/iStock.)

As adults, students need to be spoken to—not at. You will need to show them respect to ensure you receive respect back; you must treat them with dignity and value them as human beings. This simple but important attitude can make a difference in the lives of students who come from dysfunctional families, struggle with self-identity, and may have low self-worth. When students know you care and are willing to listen, they are more apt to share what their obstacles are. They may even ask for additional guidance or at least be interested in your ideas on how they might improve their behavior. However, don't be overzealous in your quest for all students to come running to you for advice—simply be present with them in case they have questions. Also remember that you may not have all of the answers; know when to get help with an area that is outside your expertise.

Traits of Other Behaviors

Though there is no official list of the various traits seen in a class, there are some common threads that consider the different personalities your students possess. Often these traits emerge later in class, after the students (and you) have shown you their best side. While students are trying to see how far you will go, or whether or not you actually enforce policy, they are also sizing up the opportunity to see what they can get away with. This is not to say every student it trying to misbehave, but rather there are other behaviors that can interfere with learning just as much as disruptive behaviors. These "traits" can easily be disguised even from your best students, but still warrant further exploration. The following five traits can be found in all students, from any culture, gender, age group, and regardless of their academic standing (Table 3.1).

Traits	*Displays Behavior*	*Ways to Redirect*
Know it all	Every time you mention a fact, answer a question, or share some new knowledge, they beat you to the punch. They may talk over you, agree/argue with what you say, and often come across as more knowledgeable about the subject than you are. 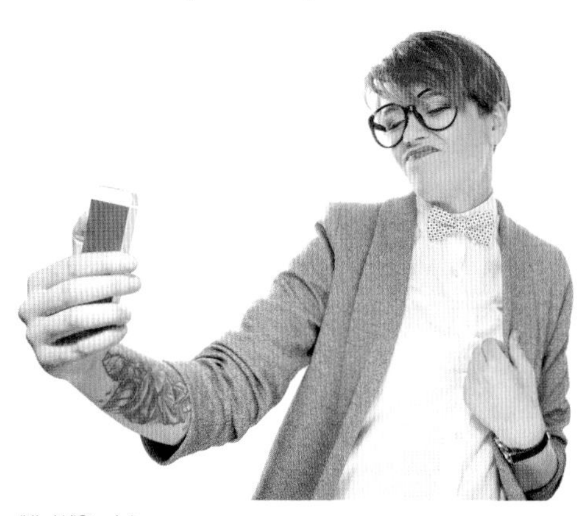 (HbrH/iStock.)	First—bite your tongue. Trying to outwit, outsmart, or argue with this student will result in that tug-of-war of the wills—and you won't win. Acknowledge them, what they have to say, and if appropriate, confirm they are right. Later pull them aside and point out that while they are obviously quite knowledgeable about the subject, others in the class are not. You'd prefer that these other students come to know the material just as well, and you need time to direct this. Also note, however, that when no one in the class wants to answer, this student may end up being your go-to person—at least they will have an answer!

Traits	*Displays Behavior*	*Ways to Redirect*
The quiet one	No matter how many questions you ask, there is no response. They are shy, quiet, soft spoken, or simply disengaged. You aren't quite sure, as they won't tell you despite various ways in asking. 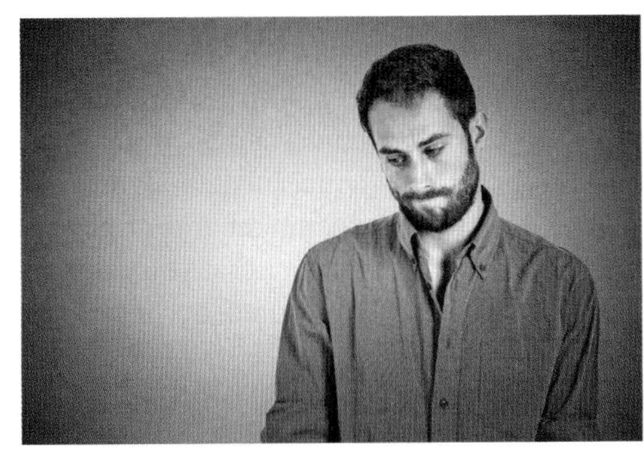 (Slphotography/iStock.)	Tough as it may be, sometimes it is best to allow these students to bloom on their own. After discovering their best learning style, move activities in that direction to see if increased engagement comes about. It could be that once they are interested, they light up and become more talkative. It may also be that they are shy or soft spoken, and the best response you will get is that they are here. You can also observe them with their peers—do they behave the same way or not? If not, don't take it personally. Try to discover things that get them out of their shell, even if during independent study time, or after class in a one-to-one.
Overinvolved	Contrary to the "know it all," this student volunteers for any and everything. Regardless of whether you need the floor mopped, the whiteboard cleaned, or simply handouts passed out, they are your personal jack-in-the-box jumping up to help. 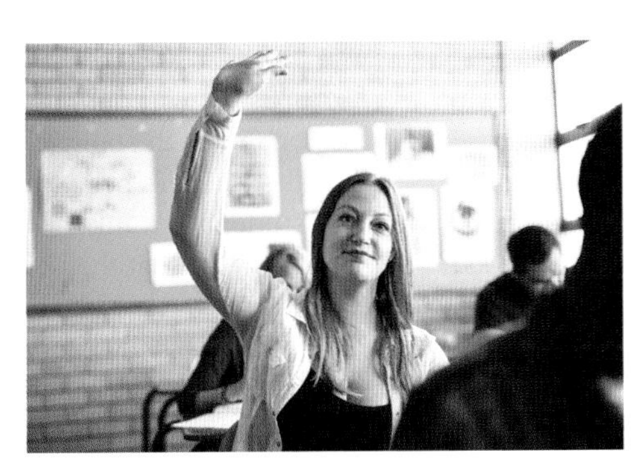 (LumiNola/iStock.)	As wonderful as this sounds, it is not a good idea to have one helper do all the work. Your class is a community of people, everyone needs to pitch in. Be certain to show respect and gratitude for this student, but also point out that you have a number of other students who need to take turns as well. As with the "know it all," you have a go-to person when no one else volunteers, but don't abuse this gift.

Traits	*Displays Behavior*	*Ways to Redirect*
Teacher's pet	They don't know the answers, nor are they overinvolved, but they do want to be your favorite. They may try to bring gifts, compliment you, or side with you on discussions. They want to be your best ally, even if you don't really have favorites. 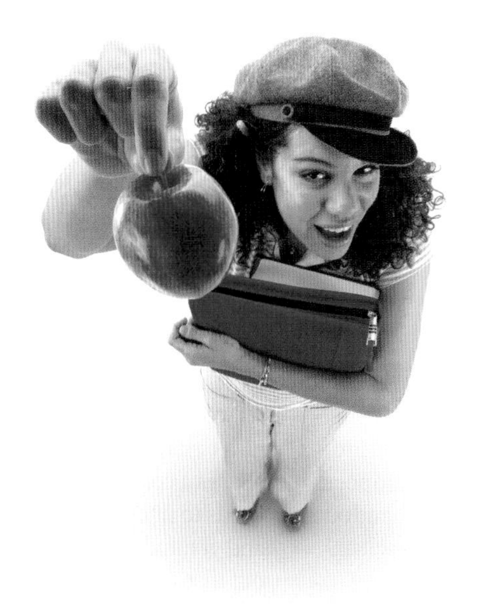 (junial/iStock.)	Warning Will Robinson! While this student's intentions may be very honorable, you could be set up for discrimination, if not by this student, by others. Absolutely never treat one student any different from how you would treat any other student. Follow policies regarding gifts, offering rides to field trips, or other measure that could be construed as personal preference. If you are concerned about any retaliation, be sure you document and/or have a witness to support the fact that you care for all students equally and do not accept bribes.
Just trying to pass	These students have a mantra: "Have pity on me, my plate is full and I'm just trying to pass." They may not always follow rules, are often the ones who try to discuss their way out of deadlines, and may even have a really good reason for not adhering to policy. They ask to be the exception and will share every reason in the book as to why they deserve to be passed. 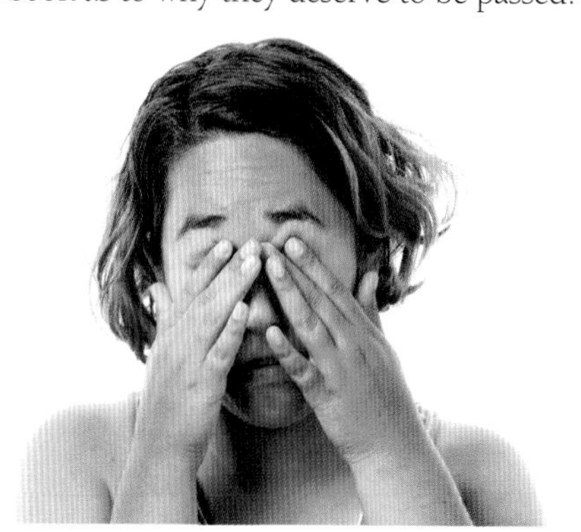 (drbimages/iStock.)	Consistency without regard to the individual personality is the only way out of this. Much like the teacher's pet, you must not allow this student to think they can obtain special treatment, or that their circumstances provide more wiggle room than others. They are entitled to what everyone has and must be held to the same standard. They are not exempt for any reason—no excuses. If you provide them with anything else, "just this one time," you will find that the ball of yarn never stops unraveling.

Reason Why They (Mis)Behave

We have mentioned the fact that you are not students' parent, but that it can be helpful to consider how the student was raised. Students who act out may have no concept that their behavior is inappropriate; students who talk back, are sassy, or what is commonly referred to as snarky may have been encouraged to speak freely. Different cultures see communication differently. Consider this reversal: in the South, it is expected that you refer to your elders as "ma'am" and "sir"; this is also true of the military when speaking to people with authority. These references are said with respect, as a sense of status. However, some people see "ma'am" and "sir" as a continuation from slavery. They consider such references as demeaning; in their eyes, we are all equal and no one outranks another regardless of age or position.

Whether or not you realize it, your own upbringing will come into play a great deal when you look at your expectations. This can be a foundation from which to have discussions about expectations, as you share why you feel the need to expect students to behave a certain way. You can start this discussion with the fact than in your generation, your culture, or how you were raised, certain behaviors were a sign of disrespect. You can ask the class to share their personal cultures and expectations and see where differences and commonalities are present. Some people think it is common sense to behave a certain way, based on their upbringing. However, as we all have come to realize, sense is left to personal interpretation, which is not always common. From this standpoint, you can ask those students (privately) who are not in compliance why they are not following the rules and why they choose to behave this way. Answers will vary greatly, but one thing is for sure: until you discover why they are not in compliance you will not be able to get their agreement, and thus, they will not adhere to the rules. Another aspect to consider is that it is possible, for whatever reason, they either see no value in the rules, don't care about the consequences, or are not motivated to adhere to the guidelines.

Once you have reviewed your expectations, understand their expectation, and have an idea of a common ground, you must be very clear on the consequences and follow through. If you are not consistent in following up with consequences, you have lost the battle before the argument begins. If your consequences are of no consequence, you will have a difficult time motivating anyone. Consider again the student who doesn't need high praise but appreciates your one-to-one tutoring. The same is true for negative consequences. You may make them stay after class as a form of making up for their tardiness, but if they couldn't care less about staying after class, you will not alter this behavior. Refer to our discussion about behaviorism in Chapter 1; this is where the positive or negative consequence must change the behavior. Unless you understand what motivates them to change their behavior, you will continue to lose in the battle of wills.

Occasionally you may find that students honestly do not know they are misbehaving or are not following your expectations. They mean no disrespect and are frankly trying to do their best. In these situations, it might be helpful to gain another person's perspective to ensure you are not unconsciously acting biased. A trusted fellow faculty member, or if it is appropriate, other students, can offer validation on the behavior or render another perspective. It is important to ensure you are not singling out any students and accusing them of misbehaving if no one else sees their behavior as inappropriate. This is another opportunity to meet with the student and review your expectations, as well as your perspective. Perhaps the student did not think that it was rude to blurt out the answer, but you would rather students take turns or raise their hands (which you have mentioned already several times in class). While this expectation is not a hard and fast rule, it does affect the dynamics of the classroom and *your* behavior. Reminding the student that you feel it interrupts the energy of the class, and that you appreciate their contribution but would prefer they raise their hand, or allow others to speak in addition, brings the behavior into light with a positive perspective. This can also be seen in the earlier table regarding the various traits—these students may not realize the behavior is unwarranted, undesired, and though not necessarily against the rules, not in alignment with your expectations. On occasion, you may also have to consider the battle and determine whether it is worth the fight. Though it is not encouraged to allow students to disobey the rules or shrug off expectations, you can spend all your energy on minor infractions which can consume your energy and focus. There is a time to simply let it go.

How to Motivate (Remember Internal/External Rewards)

In addition to being consistent, it is good to know what is meaningful to your students. The example of praise not being a motivational factor, but one-to-one time being more meaningful shows that students often appreciate your attention as the reward for their behavior. Before you consider any behavior childish, remember that adults have both internal and external motivation. While their internal motivation could be to feel good about themselves, having private time with you validates this feeling better than giving outward praise. Perhaps they have good self-esteem and were raised with plenty of praise, but their parents were always busy. Having one-to-one time could show a greater sign of respect, seeing them as an adult, and instills the fact that they are on track. Some students may have come from an environment where they felt hopeless and have only enrolled to prove they are a failure. Outward praise would be seen as insincere and therefore not effective. However, during one-to-one time, your attention and encouragement brings forth hope; the fact that you believe they can do the work may ignite a belief that had previously been snuffed out.

Reward the behaviors you want repeated. As simple as this sounds, it can be a guessing game for your students to figure you out. Be obvious with your rewards, not sarcastic or belittling, but sincere. If (for the first time ever) all students arrive on time, pleasantly reflect on this to the class and say something encouraging, like "Wow—I see everyone is here on time today. Thank you; this is really important to me. It shows that you really value my time." Students will be hard pressed to argue that you felt touched by the fact that they simply followed the rules and met the basic expectation.

Motivate the Motivators

Chances are, regardless of the size of your class (unless it is really small) there will be a few cheerleaders, one or two spokespersons, and at least one teacher's pet in your class. Use this to your advantage; have these bundles of positive energy breed more positive energy. You may do it outwardly, such as asking them to create a list of fun things the class would like (then determine if you have the resources); they may do this unofficial assignment with the class at large, or you can do it one-to-one privately with each student. For these motivators, you have stroked their ego (thereby infusing more positive energy in them) and utilized their strength to commune with their peers. Based on this mini-research project, you should know at least five things that the class enjoys doing. If you can, continue to allow these motivators to check in with the other students to ensure you are staying on track. It gives them an unofficial capacity to remain positive and validates that they are good at what they do. It cannot be stressed enough, however, to not allow this project to be seen as favoritism. You should announce to the class that you have given these students permission to ask some questions, but anyone is welcome to come to you directly. Students have permission to not respond, or to join in if they desire, but the focus needs to be on what the class enjoys as a whole. Of course, it must be realistic, such as potlucks, field trips, and guest speakers, not a ditch day or a week of no homework. You might be surprised with the ideas they come up with; the best part is, not only did you not have to invest your creative energy, but these are the "right" answers as to what motivates your students.

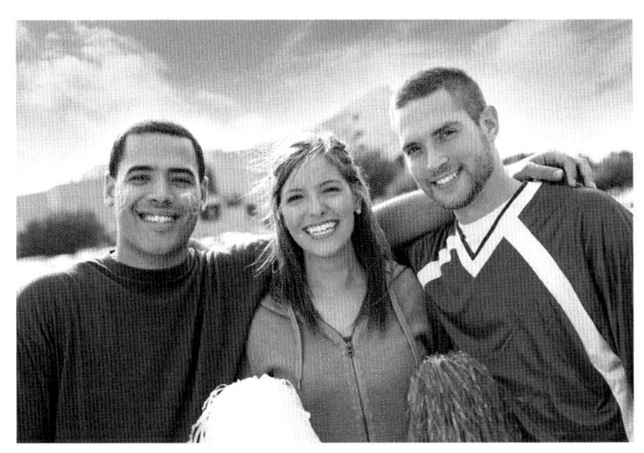

(SDI Productions/iStock.)

What to Do About Other Student Behaviors

The previous list of traits is not all inclusive; there are other traits, personalities, and behaviors that may be mixed in your class. There are the "drama queens," where everything is a big deal and everything is about them; there are the "nerds and geeks" who are only interested in the logical portion of class and seemingly don't care about anything non-tekkie, the "class clown" who wants to make fun of everything and everyone, and there are those who simply want (or need) all of the attention—however, these labels will prevent you from looking at students as they are, and if there is indeed a problem. As faculty, we must accept the numerous personalities and traits that students possess and use our own intuition and radar to ascertain what is a real problem, what is simply how/who they are, and what is superficial.

Some behaviors need immediate attention, some need no attention, but all should be monitored. If any student, regardless of their gender, age, or culture, is acting inappropriately, out of character, or is on your radar—listen to that intuition. If a student comes in late, acting boisterous, their words are slurred, and their eyes are glassy, you cannot assume they are high or intoxicated. Based on your institution's policy, you may be able to request a drug screen or ask that they speak with your manager or department head. The main point is that you speak to the behavior, not the student. It is absolutely not permissible to accuse a student of being drunk or high; indeed, this student may have a medical condition that results in this behavior. It is, however, certainly acceptable and encouraged to address the following problems: tardiness, interrupting class, and your concern for their physical health. As you are not here as their physician, and have no lab tests, you cannot diagnose what the problem is—only that you have a problem. Focus on the correcting behavior and ensure other students do the same; students should never accuse their peers of illicit behavior and need to be aware that you won't tolerate rumors. This course of action will promote a safer, albeit legal environment, where no one is pointing the finger at another and all students know their classroom is a place where they are accepted. Remember, the behavior may not be acceptable, but the student is.

Some students seem to come with a label of "problem student" invisibly etched on their foreheads. For whatever reason they come to class with a variety of issues, depending on the day. There may not be any consistency with the same problem, but each day offers a new adventure as to how they are behaving. Often these students have other issues at home and are struggling with managing their life at home and at school; it could be they live in a violent domestic situation or an emotionally abusive situation. They may fear retaliation or may feel they have no safe place to be. Some students may also have a very low self-esteem and feel that they are not worth an intervention. Young adults especially can struggle with self-identity in their early adulthood. As we touched on in Chapter 1, Erikson's psycho-social stages of development include the stages we all go through from birth throughout our life span; the fifth step in this development, according to Erikson, is intimacy versus isolation. As the emerging adult begins to charter new territories, they can be challenged as they may not feel secure in their own skin. They are unsure of themselves, where they are going, and who will be there to accompany, guide, or help them. These students may not feel comfortable sharing this feeling, as they are delighted to finally have a sense of freedom. However, this freedom comes with a very uncomfortable notion that they are now alone. In his book *Why Am I Afraid to Tell You Who I Am?* author John Powell answers with this statement: "because if I tell you who I am, and you do not like who I am, it is all that I have" (published December 1, 1969 by Argus Communications, Boston, MA). These students do not need to be coddled or parented but do need to find themselves in a sea of the unknown. As you can imagine, this can be a very sensitive area; it is important to tread lightly and use outside resources offered by your institution or your community. Remember, you are neither their psychiatrist nor their counselor, but you can direct them to such resources if they would be helpful.

There are some situations that should not be given any leeway, such as any accusations of bullying, harassment, any student caught cheating or plagiarizing, or any other illegal activity; these behaviors must be addressed immediately and require further investigation. The terms "bullying," "harassment," and "targeting" are often used without consideration of the ramifications and can be real or can be blown out of proportion. A student who complains of another student looking "weird" at them may be ultra-sensitive, whereas a student who pushes another and refers to them as *being* weird can be guilty of assault. Again, since you are not there as the behavior police, it is important to take all accusations as simply that until more information is obtained. However, do not perpetuate the use of these terms for minor offenses; students should always be able to disregard minor nonthreatening behavior and remain professional. Faculty should do the same while also modeling civility and respect.

The same is true for cheating and plagiarizing; there is zero tolerance for these behaviors and while they require further investigation, faculty should take steps to decrease such tempting actions. Be realistic and realize that students have many resources at their disposal; they can download various writing apps, pay for test answers, hire someone to write a term paper, and share answers with other students. Even the most secure testing environment can have some integrity issues, so don't be alarmed if you hear that a student cheated. If you suspect cheating or plagiarizing, be sure to do your investigation prior to confronting any student. There are also ways to decrease cheating. When students buy a test or obtain the answers, they memorize the answer, not the question along with the answers, so it is easy to rearrange the questions and/or the answers; you can also ask a short answer question (versus multiple choice) or insert reverse true/false (if it is false, make the answer true, or what is false about this answer?). Always walk around the room during a test to ensure eyes and notes aren't wandering, and be discreet; you don't want to hover over anyone shoulder or increase anxiety for students who are honestly struggling with providing the right answer. Most catalogs will address these behaviors as well as the consequences; however, when you review expectations in your first day of class it is good to clarify that you, too, have no leniency with dishonesty.

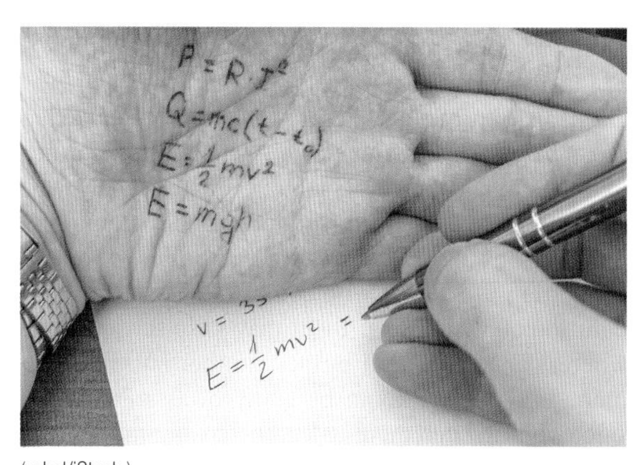

(vchal/iStock.)

Civility, Diversity, and Sensitivity

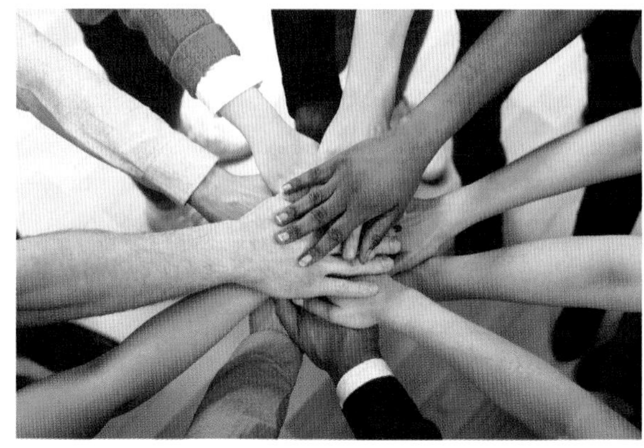
(AndreyPopov/iStock.)

Recently some new terminology has found its way into schools and the workplace as we strive to embrace all people. Being that most classes have a range of ages, religious and cultural beliefs, genders, and geographical backgrounds, faculty are faced more than ever with a new issue: how do I facilitate blending this melting pot? Civility training, diversity and inclusion, and sensitivity encompass the topics that address the variety of students we have in our classrooms. It is important to understand what these terms mean and how your institution addresses each of them. For brevity, we will touch on these terms; however, it is important to contact your manager and refer to your school catalog to ensure you are aware of what training is available and the expectation of faculty.

Diversity is the understanding that students come from diverse backgrounds, different culture and religious preferences, gender and sexual orientation, ethnicities, and span different decades in age. Inclusion is the opportunity to embrace these differences and allow them to maintain their separateness but include them all. No one is excluded or made to feel that their difference is bad or unwanted. There are no outcasts, everyone is accepted. No exceptions. Sensitivity is recognizing our difference with empathy, a connection that offers respect for who you are and what you believe in, even if it is different from my beliefs. These terms, though fairly recent, are not new to education. However, they have become more pronounced as our classes become more globally diverse and include a greater variety of backgrounds.

Other Considerations

Despite your caring heart, open mind, and calming personality, there are going to be times when your radar and intuition are right, and you need to act. If there is *any* situation whereby you or your students do not feel safe, regardless of the reason, it must be addressed. Many institutions have training on the above issues, as well as diversity, inclusion, and civility, but they also have active shooter training. As sad as it is to realize, your classroom may be a target for an angry student bent on retaliation. Do *not* attempt to address this issue on your own—you are ill equipped to do so. Always ensure that your peers know where you are, that anyone walking by your class can observe you for safety, and if you are unsafe, you have a place for you and your students to hide. Campuses prepared for this may have blinds on windows, a walkie-talkie, phone, or panic button in the classrooms. Some campuses have strolling police or security patrolling. Do not avoid these personnel—make it your policy to check in to reassure them you are safe. Ask them to walk you and your students to your car if it is late or if you have parked far away. Do not assume because you are fit, are a man, or have had self-defense training that you can handle it. Issues can quickly escalate and get out of control, no matter how much you feel you are in charge. Quite frankly, your life and the lives of your students may depend on your humility in realizing you are not in charge. Be safe—report any suspicious activity or behavior to your authorities or campus representative. As part of your orientation, find out who and where these resources are located. If all else fails, always have your cell phone charged and do not hesitate to call 911.

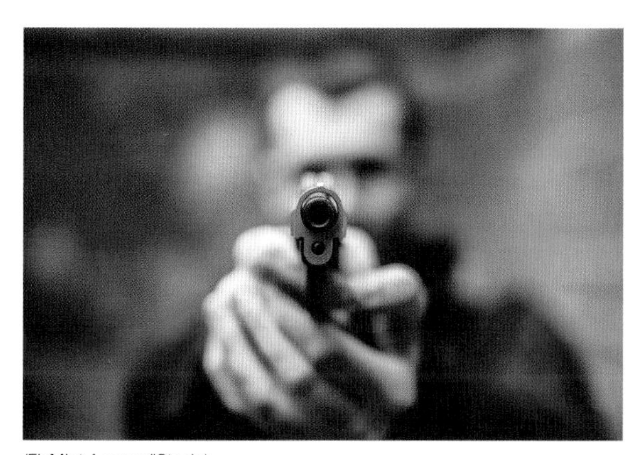

(FlyMint Agency/iStock.)

Mental Health Issues

Because students do not go through a full psychiatric evaluation prior to being enrolled, you may be faced with students who have been diagnosed with a mental illness. This can be a solitary event, such as attempting to harm themselves, or an ongoing diagnosis, such as depression or schizophrenia. Due to FERPA (the Family Educations Rights and Privacy Act; like HIPAA for health care, it preserves the rights of students in any institution receiving government funds from the Department of Education) rules and confidentiality, you are restricted in many areas and cannot speak to family or other providers without the consent of the student. Because of this confidentiality you may be in a tough spot; remember to focus on the student and their safety. If a student has confided in you that they have a medical diagnosis or mental illness, always speak privately and reassuringly to them. Try to find out who they call when they need help, and if they are seeing a physician, and whether or not they are on medication. Again, this information must be voluntarily shared by the student unless it is an emergency; without their permission you cannot contact any provider or obtain any diagnosis or history. Most mental health providers will request an informed consent by the student, and anyone you speak with on the student's behalf (such as a family member) must be on their FERPA form. There is one exception: if a student is stating that they will harm themselves or others, you have permission to contact your local police.

Developmental Issues

In addition to mental illness there are other diagnoses that may warrant your attention, such as developmental disabilities. Developmental disabilities can be physical, cognitive, or intellectual and often last throughout adulthood; common diagnoses in higher education include autism (on the spectrum), intellectual disability, or attention deficit hyperactivity disorder (ADHD). However, there are other developmental issues that can be due to trauma, a history of seizure, or other neurological functioning. Students with physical disabilities, such as being confined to a wheelchair, needing adaptive devices or braces, and the use of orthotics or prosthetics require special attention by law. These students often express their disability upfront and request Americans With Disabilities Act (ADA) services. Your campus is required to have an ADA representative; they will request paperwork and forms to be completed and will process the packet according to your campus policy. Most likely, you will be informed of the accommodations necessary for your student, such as being close to the front of the class, allowed extra time for testing, or possibly additional tutoring. While it is important to quietly honor such requests—it is not necessary to point out that these students are any different from the rest of your class. In fact, when discussing inclusion, this population suffers greatly from *lack* of inclusion, or by people only noticing their differences. These students may have been ridiculed, laughed at, or made fun of; they may feel that no one understands, and they struggle with this isolation.

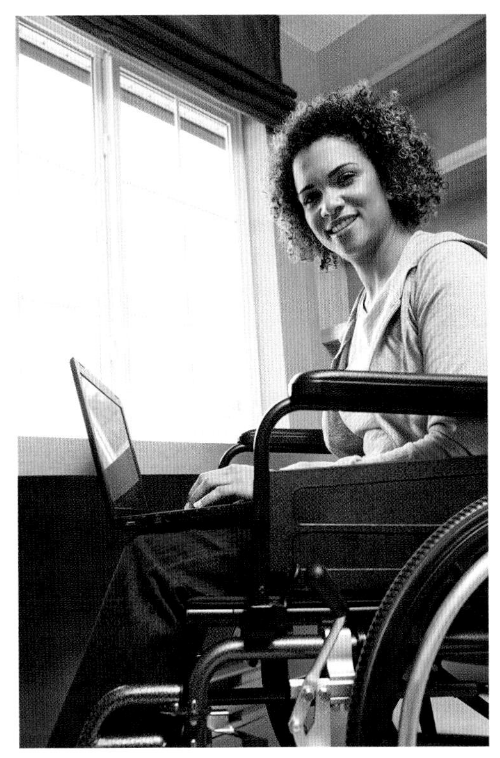

(XiXinXing/iStock.)

Fostering Empathy

As much as classroom management focuses on diversity, inclusion, and sensitivity, it is not always going to be a happy circle of students singing *Kumbaya*. There will be friction, disagreements, and students who do not appreciate respecting differences. Scheduling activities that foster empathy and allow students to connect will help everyone to "fit in." These activities can also be rooted in team building, can be self-reflection exercises, or can be integrated with other curriculum assignments. The focus should be more about how alike we are than about how different we are and how we each need to know we are valued and accepted, just as we are. If you feel it is appropriate, there are several songs, from various genres that can help break the ice and initiate discussion about how people feel when they are judged. Some suggestions are Mark Willis' *Don't Laugh at Me*, and Everlast's *What It's Like*; you can also assign this as homework and ask students to bring in songs from their favorite genre. Students don't have to love one another, or be best friends, but they do have to treat one another with respect and dignity. Outside speakers or short videos can also be a springboard for additional discussions; finding a common denominator where all students can get behind a cause or moving story can bring students closer.

Conflict Management

It will happen; students will argue, they may take it out on one another or even you. They cannot see the other person's point of view regardless of how many activities you have them do or how much you ask them to share. Don't take it personally—despite the fact it feels personal. Focus on their behavior—are they acting defensive? Are they trying to protect their own feelings? Why do they feel they need to protect themselves—are they getting singled out? Are others being rude or insensitive? Perhaps they have mistaken other people's behavior and feel that they are the subject of ridicule or can't seem to get along with others. Try to look at it with a wider lens; is their personal interpretation askew? Are you able to observe defensive posturing in others or do you honestly see these students being singled out? Is the student making more of an issue than what you can see? Remember the saying: we create our own reality. Perhaps things are not as horrible when you observe the class; instead of negating the student's perception, gently let them know that your perception is different. Again, focus on the behavior and whether the conduct is against the rules or expectations of the institution.

The same is true for faculty. If a student argues with you, thinks you are not doing your job, and challenges you, don't take it personally and don't get defensive. These students often need more compassion and lash out at the closest and safest thing they can find: their teacher. However, as mentioned earlier, no one, not even the most caring faculty member, should tolerate any physical, emotional, or other abuse. If your student's anger escalates, it's time to get help.

How to Get Back on Track

When there is an argument, altercation, or conflict, be sure to offer respect to all parties. No one should be reprimanded for saying how they feel, even if they disagree. While it is expected that students discuss their disagreements and frustrations appropriately in a respectful manner, each side needs to be heard. If your class gets disrupted and you need to address a situation, be patient and offer a listening ear—but don't get too sidetracked. These situations can easily get off track and derail the rest of day, sometimes without your awareness. More often than not, the best recourse is to allow the class to also listen and offer their perspective. You will know what is best based on how your students are able to deal with discord. When listening, also remember that silence can be the most powerful tool you have. By the mere fact that you listened attentively, you may have resolved the main issue—the need for attention. Be sure to close any discussion with equanimity and reassurance that the conversation will remain as confidential as possible.

When to Get Help

If you must deal with conflict on a regular basis, or if outbursts continue to interrupt your class, it's time to take things to the next level. You may have to speak individually with students, or with a small group after class, and let them know that their combined behavior is hurting the overall success of the class. You may want a witness present or a scribe to take notes. You may even have a contract for students to review that reinforces your expectations (based on the institution's Code of Conduct policy) and that should they behave poorly again, the consequences will ensue (list them accordingly). Including a copy to your Dean or Campus President will add additional validity that you are serious about their infraction and are supported in the process. Students will rethink their behavior if they feel that they can get kicked out of college or may suffer financially from being dismissed. While you should never threaten these consequences, you can remind them that they enrolled to be educated and reach their goals—surely this behavior was not one of their goals, and in fact, is preventing others from reaching their goals.

If you feel that you need additional help, consider having a social worker or guidance counselor come to your class. Many institutions have online resources or a hotline for such issues; they can also have a representative come to your class and speak generally about conflict, behavior management, and civility. Various free resources are also available online, especially with respect to certain groups, such as LGBTQ (lesbian, gay, bisexual, transgender, and questioning [or queer]), veterans, and those with learning or other disabilities. As we continue to expand our global classroom, we need to be sensitive to the differences and commonalities we share.

Spiritual Help and Counseling for the Teacher

More often than you may realize, you will need additional help on a more personal level. Though you may have high ideals for yourself and your students, you must temper that with reality. Not every day will be like Maria von Trapp, singing on the hillside with happy students. As we have touched on, you are entitled to get frustrated, feel overwhelmed, and may need some encouragement yourself. Regardless of your religious or spiritual affiliation, there are other principles that can offer simple guidance, such as 12-step programs (indeed we are powerless over students and cannot control them), meditation and mindfulness (such as with Zen and Buddhism), and private counseling.

Whether you practice mindful meditation, talk with a counselor, or have an outside support group, make sure that you have a place where you can share these personal feelings. While your family may be supportive, they often have their own judgments and may not be the best sounding board. Be sure your resources are positive, uplifting, and nonbiased.

Comic Relief for the Stressed-out Teacher

Try as you might, there will be days when you come home wondering why you ever thought you wanted to be a teacher. You may feel your class is off course, you are drained, and no intervention is working. While you have your resources and mentor to share with, it is important to remember that:

a. You are human and have human feelings.
b. You are *not* Wonder Woman or Superman (even they have feelings).
c. This is not your fault, but it is your responsibility. While you cannot control the outcome, you can contribute to the process.

Most of all, others have been there and have survived—sometimes with professional help, sometimes by putting it back into perspective, and many times with some comic relief. Comic relief can come from a variety of sources, a cartoon, a song, a TV series, or even another faculty member or student. It allows us to make fun of ourselves and laugh at silly things. While it is never acceptable to make fun of others, we can often make fun of the situation without any harm. The point is to keep it in perspective and realize it is a way to decrease stress. Many faculty members enjoy making fun of their situation by dreaming of winning the lottery ("would I actually leave my job if I did?") or by pretending they can say things normally not allowed. Many Pinterest, memes, and other cartoons allow simply that—a chance to laugh at our profession without anyone being hurt in the process. In the early 1970s a skit was performed by the group Cheech and Chong titled *Sister Mary Elephant*. This skit portrays a substitute nun trying to gain the attention of a school group of boys, without much luck until she yells "shut up." While most teachers understand that yelling, and saying "shut up" are not permissible, there is some comic relief in the fantasy of allowing yourself to share frustrations, and students actually being receptive to hearing this. Allowing yourself time to laugh at your mistakes, realize you're human, and knowing when to (and when not to) take a stand can help you gain better control over class and your classroom management than anything else. Above all else remember don't sweat the small stuff.

Journal: Self-reflection

1 What are my expectations of class, students, and myself?

a. My expectations of myself:

____

____

____

____

____

____

____

____

____

____

b. My students' expectations of class/me/their learning experience:

c. My institution's expectations of class/me:

2 Observations: in watching my class (or another class) what have I observed among students? When do they seem more relaxed or comfortable in their activity or learning?

3 What are some methods I will use to motivate my students?

4 What life experiences do I already have in my toolbox to deal with classroom management?

5 How will I deal with the following?

a. Conflict management:

b. Developmental or intellectual disabilities:

c. Accusations of bullying, harassment, or targeting:

d. Mental illness:

6 What are some ways I will foster empathy, inclusion, and sensitivity? List at least five specific activities you will use:

7 What resources do you have to help you with classroom management?

8 What sources are available (or will you make available) to help you with your own sense of positivity, such as spiritual help, mediation, or counseling?

9 What resources do you have for stress relief or comic relief?

10 Consider the following attitudes teachers (or any professional worker) may have:

Chicken Little or Henny Penny	The sky is always falling, and we must take shelter! Doomsday is coming and we must get prepared.	This faculty member always fears the worst, never believes anything is as good as it could be, and never feels satiated. They live in fear and worry a great deal. Regardless of how much they have done their class preparation, they know it won't be enough and the students will get bored.
Little Red Hen	If it is to be it is up to me—I cannot count on anyone else.	This faculty member is often an over-achiever, at the risk of burnout. They are stoic, put extra demands on themselves, don't ask for help but will want all of the accolades when a job is well done.

Captain America	Here to save the day! This superego stands for justice and has the power to make it possible.	This faculty member is over-positive and will snuff out any negativity, or oftentimes, reality. They forget to look at what needs to work and gloss over conflict. They want everyone to succeed and be happy, but sometimes miss the point.
Eeyore	Why bother? Why should I try? Everyone else is better than me. I won't make a difference.	This faculty member can be very hard on themselves, never feel they measure up, and will never admit that they are a good teacher. They are constantly looking at everyone else and offering praise, but never take credit for their own good ideas.

Which one (or two) do you most identify with? Why do you think that is? How can you overcome the negative aspect of this attitude?

____

____

____

____

____

____

____

____

____

____

11 In the early 1930s, Richard Niebuhr wrote what is now referred to as the "Serenity Prayer":

God, grant me the serenity to accept the things I cannot change,
Courage to change the things I can,
And wisdom to know the difference.

Rewrite this verse so that it works for you, in alignment with your spiritual affiliation:

____

____

____

____

____

____

____

____

12 Comic relief can be a harmless way to decrease stress. In the following space, draw, or copy/paste a cartoon, meme, or link to a YouTube video that makes you laugh, no matter how bad your day is:

13 The entertainment industry has many movies, songs, and other material that can be used to help you and your students understand how to deal with differences. Write down some resources that you may use for yourself and/or your class (several examples have been given—feel free to add them to your toolbox if they resonate with you):

____
____
____
____
____
____
____
____
____
____

Take it easy, take it easy,
Don't let the sound of your own wheels drive you crazy
Lighten up while you still can
Don't even try to understand
Just find a place to make a stand and take it easy
"Take it Easy," The Eagles

Chapter 4

Student Engagement

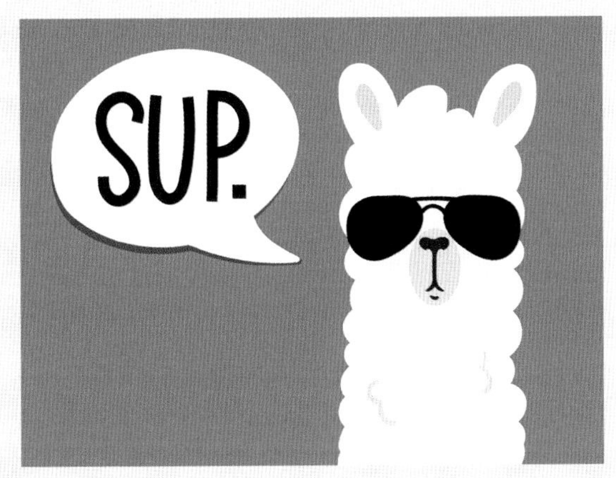

(Larysa Amosova/iStock.)

Research has shown that laughter can reduce stress, decrease one's blood pressure, help us lose weight, and in fact, help us learn. When a task is enjoyable, not only do we *want* to learn it, we also have fun doing it and will be able to recall it with more ease. It is not an oxymoron to have fun in the classroom or to be fully engaged while learning a new subject. In fact, it can take less effort and energy when the learning is enjoyable. Considering the learning theories we discussed in Chapter 1, motivation is a key element in active learning and can help even the most resistant learner gain new insight when they find the task fun. According to Csikszentmihalyi's theory of flow, when a person is fully engaged in an enjoyable task, their attention is immersed to a point where they may not even realize they are doing the task. This has been more commonly referred to as *being in the zone*: enjoying the activity so deeply that it becomes your entire focus—your world, if even for a short time.

In today's environment, despite the fact that students are guided and taught by their faculty member, students must still have the motivation, interest, and ability to carry out some of the learning on their own; they must actively participate in the learning process. As we have already touched on, this form of learning is considered *active* learning, whereby the student is engaged in the activity and has a responsibility in their learning. This chapter will review student engagement, which brings the first two chapters into a bit more focus—how do I get my students to learn through motivational techniques so that they find the learning fun and want to do more? Active learning is quite different from passive learning, where the teacher leads all learning according to preset curriculum objectives. As we move forward from understanding learning theories, planning for your course, and understanding classroom management, we get further into active learning and how to help students be engaged in the classroom. Student engagement is not only a hot topic in education, it is also the crux of active learning. In fact, if students are not engaged, then active learning won't take place (and vice versa).

Active learning demands that students become part of the learning process through a sense of discovery, wonder, enticement, or basic curiosity. When students are aroused by the subject matter and/or activities involved, they become more engaged and thus responsible in their learning. They are not only interested in participating but also become stakeholders in their own educational journey. The result is an increase in internal motivation on behalf of the student and the faculty member, as well as a more robust learning experience. It can also take less time out of the instructor's day as the "learning" seems to take on an energy of its own. Before we discuss ways to engage, we need to set the scene.

Creating Enticement

Imagine a bountiful buffet of your favorite food, carefully selected by a chef who knows exactly how you like your food, artistically displayed on an elegantly decorated table, full of bright colors and incredible designs, prepared according to whatever diet you follow—keto-friendly, low fat, kosher, lactose or gluten free ... however you enjoy your most desired foods. Absolutely no guilt, just sheer enjoyment. You would want to sit and savor every bite for as long as possible, consuming each morsel and wanting the taste to linger as you relish each bite. Although it may seem silly, think of your course the same way—you are creating a bountiful table of information, wanting each piece to be relished and the enjoyment to linger. You would want your students to be satiated, but never fully satisfied, as you want them to come back for more. While you may not create every morsel to be as tempting as the next, you can entice their appetite and lure them to at least come to the table—frequently. When students are eager to come back for more and revel in their learning, they can learn effortlessly. As we reviewed in Chapter 1, various learning theories, especially those that focus on self-motivation, perpetuate this environment, where you allow students to learn as they do best, gaining full knowledge and leading the quest for more. Keep in mind that this level of expertise takes time and may be unconventional in some institutions where traditional learning has governed the classroom. However, regardless of the old ways versus new ways of instruction, you will know if you are on task when you see the feedback and results of your assessments. Just as happy as you are when you sit back and smile after a fine meal, your students will share their delight after having an invigorating class.

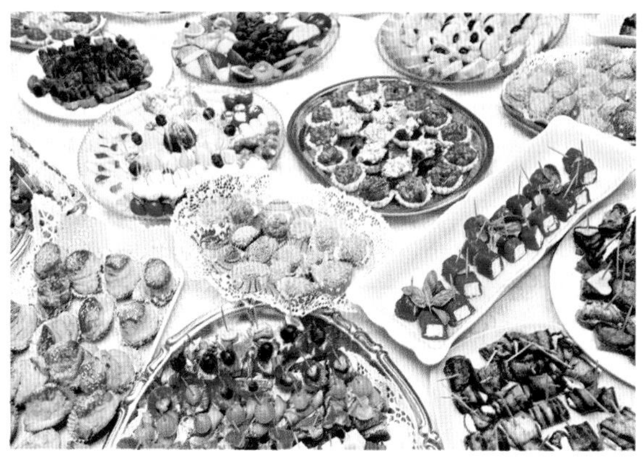

(Nastasic/iStock.)

I Scream, You Scream, We All Scream for Ice Cream!

It cannot be overemphasized how important it is to know your students, what they like, and what motivates them. If your activity is interesting to at least half of the class, there is hope. If not, you will work far harder than needed. Absolutely do not assume that everyone will love your ideas, will be interested in your activities, or will learn in this way. As previously mentioned, students learn a variety of ways. Consider ice cream—not everyone enjoys ice cream in winter; not everyone enjoys ice cream in summer either. While some like full fat, some eat only low fat; lactose intolerant people cannot eat dairy-based ice cream and may opt for soy or another alternative cream-based treat. Then, of course, there are other frozen treats like gelato, frozen custard, sorbet, ice pops, frozen yogurt ... you get the idea. Before you think everyone would want ice cream and buy all 31 flavors, you would do your own homework. You would discover whether all of your students like this treat. How many variations would you need to meet all the dietary preferences? The same is true for active learning—not everyone likes to learn one way. Your approach needs to be as varied as the myriad of ice cream or other frozen treats.

Review of Multiple Intelligence Theory (MIT)

Whether or not you ascribe to Gardner's theory of nine intelligences, there is at least some benefit in viewing a variety of settings in which students can learn, using them as learning environments. Although you have come up with your own list, we will extrapolate on your ideas by reviewing them as an engagement perspective versus an individual learning style. In the table that follows (Table 4.1), each of the nine intelligences are listed from Chapter 1, as well as a review of how that student learns or where their strengths may be. In the third column there are a few ideas of how to use this as an engagement activity in the classroom, or how to create this type of environment. The idea is to use these for the whole class, in addition to the individual learner, to instill a more well-rounded approach. According to Gardner, we each

TABLE 4.1 **Creating Multiple Environments in the Classrooms**

Intelligence	Attribute	Engagement Activities
Logical/mathematical	Good with numbers, ability to think abstractly, enjoys solving problems	• Create (or have half of the students create) experiments from the science perspective (physics, chemistry), from a mathematical perspective, or from a social behavior perspective. Have the other half perform the experiment. The creators can guide, evaluate, and offer feedback to the students doing the experiment. Then switch the roles so everyone has an equal turn. • Bring in various puzzles and create games from the puzzle. Perhaps there are behaviors associated with it, such as one person doesn't participate, or another person tries to be the boss. • Dissect things, such as parts of a body (for an anatomy class) or parts of a computer, or even a sandwich for a nutrition class. • Provide a topic in current events or controversial issue that students can analyze—some can be observers, perhaps a moderator.
Linguistic/verbal	Good with words, speaking, verbal skills	• Storytelling and small group teaching allow students to share their talents by talking. • Allow students to create or present case scenarios, complete with the what-ifs, and walk their peers through the simulation. • Use any opportunity to debate, no matter which side—have them support the opposite side from what they believe is right. • Have students create role playing scenes or skits based on the subject matter.
Tactile/kinesthetic	Good with hands-on skills, body movement	• All students need to move, so let them! Get the class out for a walk, a dance, or a chance to play a physical game. • In addition to physical movement, allow time for students to build and use their skills to create physical things (like a game or poster board or use Tinker Toys/other building sets) or rearranging the classroom for a game. • Students can also build data based projects, such as spreadsheets and reports to reflect progress on assignments completed; such spreadsheets would show how well they are doing in reaching their goals.
Aural/musical	Good with rhythm, can hear different tones	• Have students create or find songs related to the subject, or they can rewrite the words to a popular song for the subject at hand. • Put students in charge of music or poetry, according to the favorite genre, to play before class, right after break, and at the end of class. Have some guidelines, but allow them to choose how to start or end the day. • Task students with videos, infomercials, and podcast—it can even be a recording of a particularly difficult class.
Spatial/visual	Able to "see" it in their mind, good with spatial abstract context	• Students can draw pictures, create virtual visualizations, and use videos to elaborate on concepts. • Have students create posters, a collage, or use memory games to pull similar material together.
Intrapersonal/solitude	Ability to be self-aware, in tune with one's self	• Provide time and a composition book for journaling, and allow students to decorate their journal in a way that represents themselves. • Assign some activities during or after class for independent study.

Intelligence	Attribute	Engagement Activities
Interpersonal/social	In tune with others, empathetic	• Encourage students to create plays/skits or simulation activities—team up like-minded talents. • Assign exercises whereby students must interview or poll others, or obtain a history. • Provide a chance for students to be leaders or representative in a community or peer-to-peer activity.
Naturalistic/ environmental	Good with plants, animals, and nature	• As much as the weather permits, have class outside. • Use plants, animals, or other things in nature, perhaps have a plant in the classroom that grows along with your students. • As you interject issues for debate and discussion, be sure to use global issues.
Existential	Deeper awareness of self and one's purpose in life	• In addition to journaling, encourage self-reflection related to spiritual or other forms of mediation. • Invite local or globally impactful leaders to be guest speakers, or watch their talks together as a class; provide a framework for students to get out of themselves and see their passion on a bigger level with like-minded people.

possess all of these traits; it's just that some have had an opportunity to become stronger than others. Your students may even find that they become stronger in this area by virtue of having the opportunity to hone this skill or trait.

As you can imagine, there are several of these intelligences that can use the same activities. While asking your students to journal after a long day of activities, or on a controversial subject, you are tapping into their existential, intrapersonal, and verbal strengths. When you go outside and do a group activity or a team-building activity, you have intertwined naturalistic, interpersonal (or intrapersonal, based on the activity) strengths.

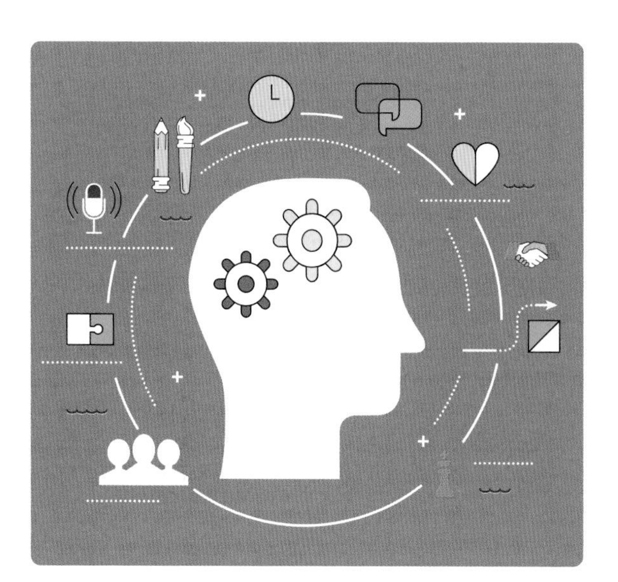

Use of Imagination

Let's face it, you will not always have the creative energy to come up with a plethora of fun activities to keep your students engaged for 5 to 8 hours straight. However, part of student engagement means that the students need to be engaged, including the creation of the activity. While you cannot simply walk into a classroom and ask for your social learner to create an activity that focuses on verbal, visual, and aural learning, you can assign a group of students (with those traits) the assignment to create a podcast, video or infomercial, or a song that encompasses something you are asking them to memorize. As you know, songs can be created from a variety of sources and inspirations and can be used for all subjects regardless of how intensive or simple they are. For example, songs have been created for cardiology (how the blood flows), to the brain (12 cranial nerves), to math (multiplication),

English (grammar), and even for civic and government classes! Many of you will recall the sing-along cartoon series called *Schoolhouse Rock*; it was instrumental in providing songs and lyrics for a range of subjects that teachers needed students to learn. This TV series became very popular with such songs as *Conjunction Junction*, *I'm Just a Bill*, and *Interplanet Janet*; it aired from the mid-1970s to the 1980s and left the airways for a short time. Due its popularity and the fact that it actually helped students learn various subjects, it was returned in the 1990s with even more subjects. Added to *Schoolhouse Rock*'s repertoire were more current issues, such as the weather and climate change, money, and environmental issues like recycling. Students can be assigned these *Schoolhouse Rock* cartoons to watch for inspiration and get their own imagination jump started. Remember to be clear on expectations (such as timing, refraining from anything vulgar, or the use of profanity) and to choose the "right" students.

The logical and solitary learners may have their imagination sparked by creating rubrics or an evaluation form. They could even be your research analysts and send surveys to determine what students enjoy the most or what additional ideas they have for a particular topic. Verbal learners are great with providing instruction, teaching a lesson, and can be the moderator for the class when activities ensue. Small groups should comprise a variety of learners so that they can ignite one another's passion and draw energy from their group, not zap the energy out of you. You simply need to set the stage, provide the assignment (and clear guidelines), and allow them to come to you for questions, guidance, and a check in to ensure they are on track.

Use of Technology

Regardless of the demographics of the student, the culture or environment of the class, or even the subject matter, almost any class can include technology as a launchpad to get students more engaged. While millennials, Gen Z, and even some Gen Xers enjoy technology, when allowed to use their phone/tablet, most students can follow along, as this "form" of technology spans across all ages, nations, and languages. Below are some activities that use technology and allow students to pull out their cell phones in order to participate. These activities can be done in groups, as an independent exercise, and can even be led by students. It takes little prep time and can fill a 20-minute lag in a lecture or a full day of teambuilding.

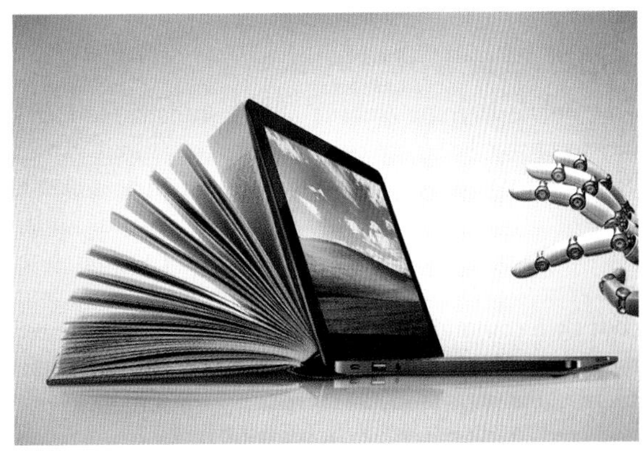

(Muni Yogeshwaran/iStock.)

When creating technology-based activities it is important to ensure a few KEY elements:

- It must be FREE—as in no charge, no subscription service, no download, and no risk of computer viruses for you or your students. Be sure to check the fine print to ensure there is no trial period with a fee or subscription later, or that you are entitled to it as an educator, but the cost is deferred to your students.
- It is *easy* for YOU to use, as well as your students. While your students may be more tech-savvy than you are, you must understand how to use the tool, have easy access, and enjoy the site. If it is not easy to navigate, or if you do not fully understand how to use the site as a tool in the classroom, move on to another site. It is imperative that you are seen as a master of this activity if you are to guide students, not as an apprentice learning as you go along.
- It is compatible with ALL smartphones, android-based phones, Mac, and Windows. If you're having students use a particular website or app to complete an assignment or to do work in small groups, it needs to work with everyone's technology. While most online games are compatible with both android and iOS, some are not. Be sure your technology-based resources are inclusive of both.

Online Games and Resources

Here are a few simple games that you can incorporate into the class; these are broad based and can cover a variety of subjects. As with any resource, be sure to review the material, as well as how to use it, long before you try to include it in your class.

QUIZLET

This online learning website allows students and faculty to create flash cards, tests, and play various games in a larger community, a small group (such as a class), or individually. There are preset games, flashcards, quizzes and other communities that students can join. You and your students can also create your own material and your own community, and you can use this to reinforce the subject(s) you are teaching. Within this site there are different ways students can study or test themselves: flashcards, multiple choice quizzes, fill in the blank, even spelling tests within your category; some subjects have diagrams and terms so that students can learn anatomical parts and functions or chemistry equations. There are games you can use to reinforce learning such as a matching game and an asteroid-like activity. By incorporating these tools, students reinforce their knowledge of simple and complex materials. These activities can be started in the classroom to ignite their interest and get them started learning the subject you are teaching and have them follow along with additional activities at home. You can also form small groups and use the activity (such as matching or fill in the blank) as a friendly competition.

POLL EVERYWHERE

Most teachers forbid the use of cell phones in the classroom; however, Poll Everywhere allows students to bring out the forbidden fruit and use it as part of their learning. Again, there are a variety of categories and subjects that parallel your own, but you will need to review them before using them in class. You can also create your own subjects and questions, especially if it's used for a test review, or as a pretest to determine what your students know before you begin teaching the class. Be careful when signing up for this, as there is a pricing matrix involved that can be confusing. In higher education it is a free enrollment; simply allow your students to work along with you.

KAHOOT!

As with the previously mentioned online games, this resource can use preset material, or you can create your own. You can create questions with multiple choice answers, ask students to respond via their cell phone, and determine how much the students understand the subject matter by their responses. The platform tallies the results to determine who has responded and how many students answered the question correctly. As with the other online games, you can do it as a large class activity or small group competition; students can also create their own games and do it as homework or bring it to the classroom to instill more critical thinking. When playing Kahoot! students can have fun but also be discreet if they do not know the answer.

JEOPARDY

Since the mid-1980s this game show has been one of America's favorite question and answer games. Students of all ages are not only familiar with the games, but its world-renowned theme song titled *Think!* Creating your own *Jeopardy* game can be a bit time consuming, but there are many advantages to this investment. The primary one is the familiarity of the game and the rules; most students know how to play, and you need no orientation. Second, once you create the game, it is there for all classes. If you create a *Jeopardy* game for an anatomy class (selecting your five or six primary systems as the categories), the material is there for every anatomy class. Tweak it if you find errors, but it stays in your toolbox. Have a general one for teambuilding, such as common facts about your college, classroom etiquette, or careers in the industry. While you become Alex Trebek, the game show host of *Jeopardy!*, your students will become more savvy in their critical thinking skills (something we will expand on in Chapter 5).

Strategies and Toys

While there are no costs for the games discussed earlier, there may be a slight cost to get the "toys" or tools needed. If you are going to use these games as a teambuilding exercise, you will need some sort of buzzer to determine who has the correct answer. While you can go in a particular order, asking each group their question one group at a time, student engagement is much higher if students can pound on a loud buzzer to show their enthusiasm and the fact that they feel they know the answer. Buzzers can be purchased at an inexpensive price or you can create your own. Again, you don't have to come up with the idea of how to make a buzzer—let your kinesthetic students build one. If you are in close proximity to other classes or a lobby, be sure to warn your neighbors that your class may be a little louder today; obviously have some flexibility if other classes are testing. If desired, have a small prize for the winners; if your budget does not cover such costs, bragging rights are equally as coveted and are free. Sometimes these rights are more valuable, as they instill self-efficacy and competence in all players.

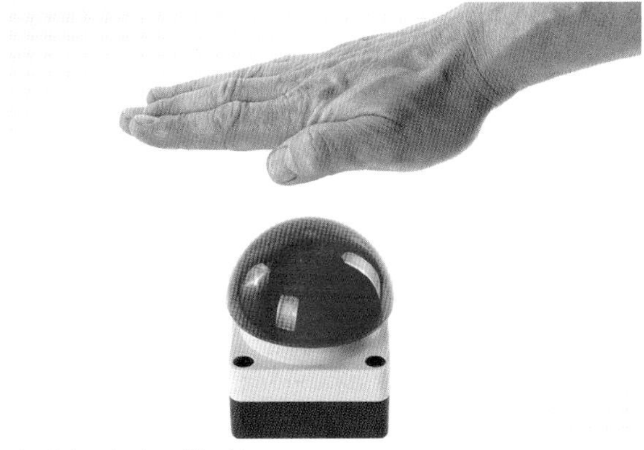

(Jan-Schneckenhaus/iStock.)

In addition to the buzzers, have the teams wear a team "uniform"; something simple like a color scheme in their regular clothes (team red, team blue) or have T-shirts they can wear over their school-based uniform. You can also allow teams to create their own T-shirt with their team slogan. If you are with this class for a longer duration or will teach multiple classes to this group, they will have more than one opportunity to use this attire. Never require students to pay for an outfit, or any tools; while it may seem inexpensive to you, many of your students may be struggling financially and should not be put in the situation of having to pay for a non-essential item. More importantly, if you choose to buy a cheap T-shirt for students to use, be sure you do so for all students. You cannot pay for only those students who cannot afford this item; be fair and be consistent.

While teams are a great way to play games, sometimes you will want to use the activities as a solitary experience. As we try to touch on all learning styles, the solitary learner who believes they are the smartest student in the class (and indeed may be) will show just how competitive they can be when they are questioned as an individual. In fact, they may think that working with a team slows them down or dumbs down the material. Be very careful not to provide an activity whereby these students take over the activity and make other students feel inadequate. If you have one or two students who truly know more than the others, allow them to be the leader of the game/activity. They will gain pride in confirming the correct answer and may even be humbled when they stumble upon a question they didn't know or get wrong. The idea is that everyone has fun and learns, not that anyone feels inferior or stupid. A word of advice: once you start using these games you may find your students asking for them repeatedly. Be sure that you are comfortable repeating this activity in various formats; showing them a game one day and never doing games again will defeat your carefully planned course. Students may also feel a sense of disappointment which can make their interest waver. Remember the idea is to increase engagement throughout their learning continuum, not just for a few days. If your peers do not know how to continue this enthusiasm and are afraid to play games, offer to guide them or share how effective it was for you and your students. No one needs to feel intimidated by technology, no matter how many times we refer to our mobile computing devices as "smart."

Virtual Reality Experience or Other Realities

While these online games may not feel too far-fetched, technology has taken education to the next level. Though some are still in their infancy, other interactive activities use technology to offer role playing in a co-op setting, taking on new personas and following a storyline or strategy; some platforms have a three-dimensional (3-D) setting whereby students can interface with a hologram and practice skills or procedures; other virtual experiences run simulations so that students can practice their profession without hurting (or killing) anyone. While it seems like something you would find in the next century (or at least the next decade), these methods of learning have been around for decades and used in such applications as aerospace engineering, the military, and medical products, such as prosthetic robotics. Though not all institutions are this tech savvy or can afford these interfaces, it is important that your students at least know of them, how they are used, and what lies in their future. After all, they will be the ones who will either be using them or working within a profession that uses them as they pursue their own careers.

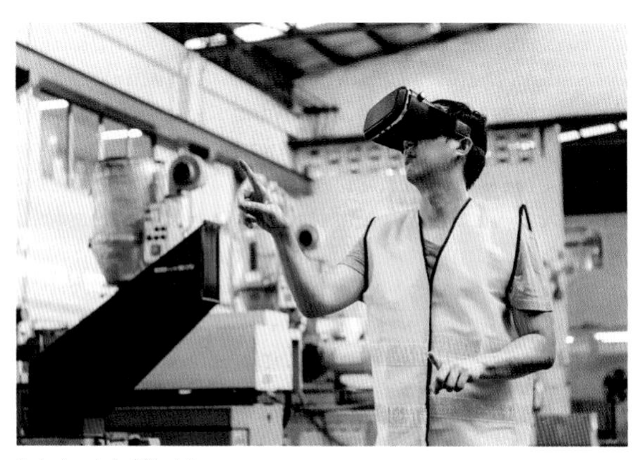

(twinsterphoto/iStock.)

In addition to your own reality and that of your students, our world has unique opportunities to join or create other realities. While some realities have stemmed from board-based games, movies, or books, there are several role-playing games (RPGs), such as *Dungeons and Dragons*, as well as massively multiplayer online role-playing games or MMORPGs. Like *World of Warcraft* and *Lord of the Rings* that students can participate in (albeit as another being or character). Many of these have a cult-like following but offer a very good opportunity to think in another dimension. Several students will already be involved in some sort of online gaming (not to be confused with gambling) and will be happy to share with you their quests, adventures, and plots to overcome another entity or territory. This may be an opportunity whereby your students teach *you*—if you are open and appear genuinely interested. Advanced thinkers may even be able to create a classroom reality, creating different characters and scenarios for the other students to participate in. This is similar to case-based scenarios but more interesting as students take on the personalities of the role. These realities/scenarios can be quite useful in professions where there are various roles who must work together in a specific situation, such as medical or nursing or security and law enforcement.

VRE or virtual reality experience is a unique learning platform that encompasses a VR (virtual reality) software program and VR interactive goggles. Students can view a simulation via the VR goggles and interact with the 3-D hologram. So, while a student is learning about history they can (virtually) explore a map and search landmarks, comparing different geographical regions from another time period in history until the present day. Medical students can attempt to perform various surgeries and sutures, without ever touching a body or cadaver. This form of education has become increasingly popular in areas where there is either a large cost (cadavers aren't cheap, but neither are human lives) or multiple layers of learning (engineering and architecture not only involve expensive supplies, but also entail other specialty areas). Using VRE, students can explore individually or together, based on the activity and how the software program is set up.

In addition to virtual reality there is the less expensive, though still interactive, augmented reality (AR). AR uses a 3-D platform and software program to interact via smartphone, tablet, or another computer device. While goggles are not necessarily involved, there are various animations and a sense that the hologram/animation is part of the current world. Consider going to a hairstylist and wanting a different color or hair style. Before your hairstylist ever shampoos your head, you can determine what you want your new look to be. Using an actual picture of your hair/head, you can "try on" different colors, various styles, and new designs to determine if you like them. Once you select the look you want on your virtual self, your hairstylist has an exact blueprint of what to do and you have a sneak preview of how you will look. This methodology is currently being used by IKEA's AR, where shoppers can select a piece of furniture without ever leaving their home. By simply using your phone (and the IKEA app), you can scan the place in your living room where you think that floral printed chair should go, choose the right floral printed chair on IKEA's app, and copy and paste it into the "virtual" spot in your living room. You can determine whether or not it matches; perhaps the chair looked better in the showcase design room but not necessarily next to your leopard skin rug. No harm done and no cost involved thanks to AR.

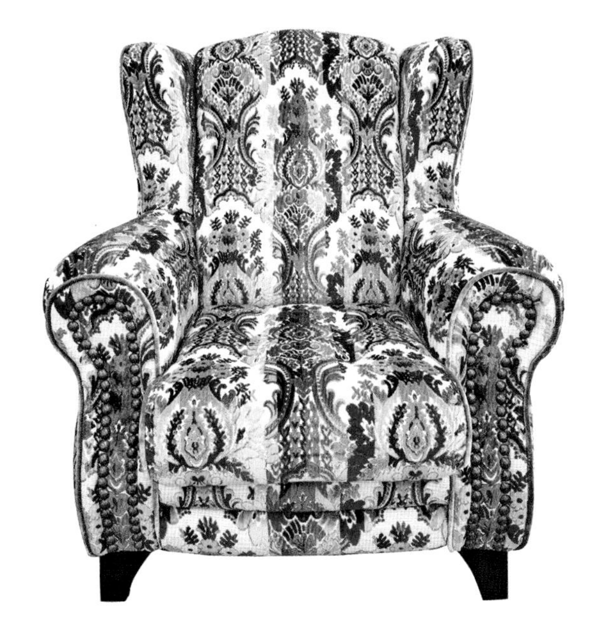

(Zozulya/iStock.)

While many of your students may be aware of AR, VRE, and RPGs, some may not. Make sure that any discussion or use of these realities begins with a baseline so everyone's interpretation is the same. Those who are more advanced can offer further information or insights, as long as they don't take over the discussion or activity.

More Games

Indeed VRE, AR, and RPGs can seem like something out of *Star Trek*; however, almost any game can be converted to an online game or interactive class activity. Based on the subject you are teaching; your peers may know some of these specialty games and have additional resources. Being that your classroom will have a variety of students from various cultures and different ages, you can take a game from the past or present and turn it into a class exercise. Below are some simple ideas; the rules are the same: learn and have fun. If a student doesn't know how to play or the class has no reference, take time to preview the games without any penalty. Maybe you will spend a few minutes covering the rules and the strategy, and then play one or two practice rounds to ensure everyone is comfortable. If some students are still uncomfortable or shy, be sure to pair them up with other students who are more comfortable and knowledgeable. As stated, you do not always have to offer prizes; the excitement from playing and the chance to boast that you won are well-earned prizes in and of themselves.

Before you feel that you are totally out of touch with any reality, it may be comforting for you to know that several games from the 1970s and 1980s have been revamped and are still popular in the 21st century (you are out of luck if you loved *Hollywood Squares*, as that left the airways in 2004). Below are some popular TV game shows that you can creatively convert to a game about anything. To make it easier for you, some examples are provided to get your creative juices flowing; remember the rules: it must be fun (and free) and students must learn something (preferably about the course you are teaching).

$100,000 PYRAMID

This game requires that students work in pairs to determine the answers compiled into a pyramid. While you are required to create the "categories," these could also be terms you want students to know. The answer needs to be clear (no other answers would work) and it should be timed.

Pros: best used for a small class, students must be able to elaborate enough to give ample clues.

Cons: if students do not know the material this will not work.

Example: consider an anatomy class: have six categories related to one system, like cardiac. The first answer/term is "heart"; the person giving the clues says, "this is the main part of the system, where blood runs through," and continues giving clues until the recipient responds. Another answer/term is "valve"; clues could include "this allows blood to come through or not and acts as a gateway; there are two main ones called mitral and tricuspid." Again, it is timed, and the clue giver cannot say the term "heart" or "valve" or they are disqualified. In a small class, you can have a few teams compete with a few onlookers. However, it is important the pace continues quickly so no one gets bored.

ARE YOU SMARTER THAN A 5TH GRADER?

Everyone's most fun and humiliating game, this professes that a fifth grader would know more than you, or that everything you learned as a child has been forgotten (as adults don't use the same materials that fifth graders learn). The game allows the participant to answer at a basic level (first grade) and proceed through a series of questions at each grade level until they reach fifth grade; the bonus next round is the million-dollar question. If they answer the question, they can go to the next level and earn points or some other reward.

Pros: this has a scaffolding effect on subjects whereby students need to know basic information but must also build on that knowledge to understand more advanced terms or concepts. This can easily be used for a test review, as long as you start with simple concepts and move on to more complex terms. Students can work as a team or as individuals, with a team support system.

Cons: because of the ladder of questioning, you will need quite a few questions to pool from to create this game. While you can employ other students to help, you would need to mix it up. For example, if everyone offered one easy question and one hard question, you could have a mix of questions to choose from to create your game. Even if the student, as a participant, got their own question, they would know just one answer; not enough to tip the scales of knowledge but be sure it doesn't offer a game winning bias.

Example: going back to that anatomy class, perhaps the overall category is skin. Questions would be: how many layers of skin do we have? Name them. In addition to the dermal layers, there are bulbs—name them. As you can determine, these questions go from simple to complex and require an "end point"; knowing the dermal layers as well as major accessory structures.

FAMILY FEUD

Again, this game is best used for smaller classes, though there can be audience participation. This game requires preparatory work as you (or your logical learners) will need to "survey" your students ahead of time or use specific textbooks or research articles to show rankings. Categories are given and results are based on the population. Students must work in a family, or small teams, to offer the best answer in order to reach the more popular results.

Pros: allows students to offer more than one right answer, encourages teambuilding.

Cons: not good for all subjects; but excellent when there is more than one right answer in a subject, such as psychology or the social sciences.

Example: in your first few weeks of class you can cover learning styles and share MIT. Having the category of "kinesthetic learner," the teams must come up with ways this student learns. While there is a top ten listing, students will want to choose the most popular answer. Having surveyed your kinesthetic learners (and reviewed your handbook) you come up with response: Survey says: hands on!

LET'S MAKE A DEAL

While there are several versions, including dressing up in eccentric costumes, the premise is to negotiate with the person from the audience to see if they can gain a prize, preferably the biggest prizes. Often these prizes are concealed, and the participant must rely on luck to choose the option (and hopefully get a better prize) or stick with what they have. A twist on this game for the classroom is to negotiate with students on their answers instead of rewarding them with prizes.

Pros: easy to use with little preparation, just requires some intuitive thinking of when to put it in your plan for the day/week. Requiring students to be prepared before class (and even to dress up ahead of time) would require more planning but could yield more creative participation.

Cons: can be limiting based on the subject matter; good for short periods or to interject when reviewing heavy material.

Example: a psychology class reviewing mental illness requires students to think of a myriad of diagnoses in the *Diagnostic and Statistical Manual of Mental Disorders,* Fifth Edition (DSM-5). While many seemingly overlap, there are distinctions for each disease. You ask a student what the diagnosis would be for a person who is showing sadness, is withdrawn, and refuses to participate in previously enjoyable activities. The student offers "anxiety" as their answer (though not the best answer), but behind door #1 is "manic-depressive," door #2 has "schizophrenia," and door #3 has "depression." Regardless of the doors chosen (or even if the student keeps their answer) they earn points, as each of these diagnoses have depression. However, the most points go to the student if they chose door #3.

WHEEL OF FORTUNE

Much like hangman, this game requires students to fill in the blank. Before they can shout out any answer, however, they must earn the right to offer a letter and must purchase vowels. Although you won't use actual money, you can use points or *Monopoly* money for students to gain a real-world perspective.

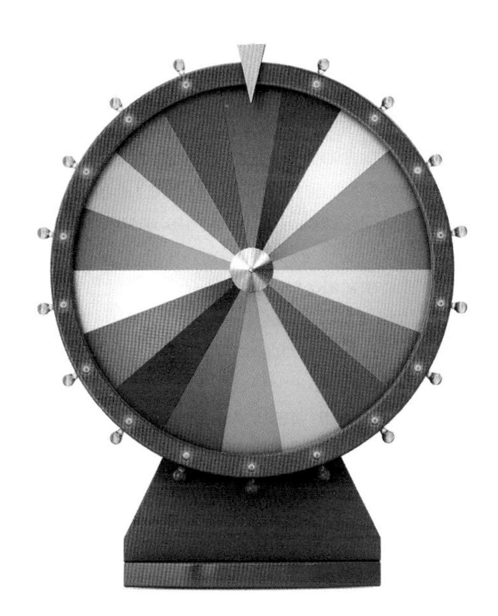

(Rost-9D/iStock.)

Pros: excellent for classes that have a lot of terms, or where spelling is important. Extremely easy to use with little preparation.

Cons: not suited for all classes and does not promote higher order thinking. Will require some sort of wheel (either handmade, purchased, or other means to offer the incentives and "money").

Example: consider a language class, such as French. You could offer a definition and put the dashes on the board for the students to fill in the blank. The student must spin the wheel to earn money and offer a letter. If your definition was "love" the student must suggest the letters "l," "m," or "r"; if they gave any other letter, they would lose whatever amount the wheel rested on. They must also have enough money to buy the vowels "a," "u," and "o"; it would be up to you whether you would provide the apostrophe or not for l'amour, which is the French word for love.

More Ideas

This is a small sampling, as any game can be turned into a fun activity to review course material. Even popular reality TV shows, as *Survivor* and *Judge Judy*, can be morphed into a class activity. Before you start your own rendition of *The Voice* or *Dancing With the Stars* be sure you have a goal in mind; remember, the learning needs to pertain to the subject matter at hand (unless the purpose is for teambuilding). You also need to make sure you have a practice run at home or with other non-students. If you are too embarrassed to incorporate other human beings, your pets may be eager to sit there and pretend with you. At least you will have a chance to do a practice run without much embarrassment (and Fido will never tell on you). Though the Internet, your friends, and your students may have more ideas—remember the KISS principle: keep it simple and *sweet*.

Discussions and Debates, Not Didactic

Some engagement activities require less preparation, but still require a great deal of participation. Debates and discussions can be formal, as previously mentioned regarding controversial subjects, or can simply be included on basic topics, like care of the elderly or nutrition. For example, you could ask your students to do a literature review on the most common signs of elder abuse or the top trending diets. A discussion can be held on what could be done about elder abuse, the fragmentation and depersonalization that some institutions create, and how sometimes abuse may not be abuse at all. The nutrition class can offer pros and cons on each diet, while others bring in (or create a sample, collage, or poster) foods included in each diet. In both these examples there is ample room for discussion, as varying cultures, ages, and personal experience can offer different perspectives. These topics can incorporate higher thinking such as moral, ethics, and values, and can roam into other subjects such as sociology, world-based medical care, and global nutrition.

In these examples, the faculty member is either part of the audience or the facilitator. The focus is to allow the students to explore these topics based on their own ideology and values; you may play devil's advocate if you find everyone on the side of the argument or in total agreement. Another example is in the discussion of euthanasia; while some students may feel that people who are suffering, are elderly, or have been diagnosed with a terminal disease have the right to determine when they die, these same students may be hard pressed to agree to such actions for mentally ill patients, who have the same suffering. Students must be able to discuss matters openly, without judgment, and be reassured that all answers are acceptable. These decisions are very personal and cannot always fall into right or wrong categories; you can, however, use this as an opportunity to cover legal obligations and the restraints of the law according to both state and federal jurisdictions.

Virtual Class Discussions

If you teach online, don't think that the face-to-face classrooms have all the fun. Online discussions offer as much creativity, although it may not be in real time. You must be more engaged with your students and often meet outside of class time to prepare these activities, but it can be done. You can also use virtual meeting rooms, such as Zoom, WebEx, and Skype to have an interactive class. These sessions are a bit different if everyone is joining from their living room but can even be more fun as you see folks in their pajamas (maybe you even have that as a requirement). The idea is to get the students to where you want them to be, to make learning fun, and to build on prior knowledge.

Personal Experience

As we have discussed ways to use outside influences to engage the student, there is nothing better than personal experience to get a conversation going. Different than debates and discussions, this has a particular reference point and usually is from a specific perspective. When studying chemical dependency, for example, you may have an outside speaker come and share their story (either as an alcoholic, an addict, or one who has lived with an addict). They may share how they felt, their significant other's involvement and impact, how they eventually got help, and how they are staying on track or staying sober. You can ask members of the student audience to share any personal reflections, questions, or their own story if they feel comfortable. Chances are that you will have at least a few students who have experienced this disease or been affected by it; to be safe, you may have some students prepared with questions that you have created just to get the sharing started.

These resources are often discovered by asking your peers or circle of friends for a reference. If you cannot find an appropriate source this way, you can search online for local community groups; if possible, go to one of their meetings to listen to how this person would speak, the basic principles of the program, and whether they are open minded toward students. Some programs (or people) are very focused on the principle that there is only one way of life and will preach to students instead of sharing their own experience. Also be sure that there is no charge for the speaker coming to your class; let your institution know you will have an outside speaker (see Chapter 2 for more detail). If your speaker is a close friend or other faculty member, make sure students honor anonymity and confidentiality. While this person is willing to share their personal story, they may not be ready to broadcast and tweet their life to the world quite yet.

Flipping the Classroom

Flipping the classroom has not only become a buzz phrase and a way of teaching, there also are now companies that specialize in this tactic. This instructional strategy and method, though not new, uses the concept that students can and should direct their learning instead of the teacher doing all of the teaching. By flipping the classroom so that students are directing the learning, faculty can resume their roles of mentor, guide, and facilitator. This technique can require just as much planning and oversight as another class, as some students may take off on tangents or incorporate other discussions not appropriate for the subject matter.

When considering this technique, start with what you want your student(s) to do and what the objective is. If the objective is for you to take a break from teaching, you need to rethink your strategies. Chances are you have spent too much time lecturing and not enough of the class time allowing and using students to discover material on their own. Review the earlier ideas and determine which ones suit your style best. If the objective is for your students to work better in groups, be clear on your expectations and don't make them too high. While teamwork is important in every profession, they may still have differences that they are not mature enough to overcome yet. If the objective is actively learning and student engagement (the correct answer!), you still need to temper this with when it is appropriate *not* to flip the classroom. After all, you are the teacher.

Don't Flip Out!

There is actually a time to not flip the classroom, such as if there is fairly new material that you must cover in a short amount of time, or a review for a test that many students have not yet mastered. Asking other students to lead the review or cover unchartered territory in a crunch can leave everyone frustrated and may even cause errors. Just as you need time to plan a class, any student or group of students presenting will need time to plan an activity; in fact, they may even need *more* time as they are not as used to teaching as you may be (even if this is your first class). If you are having a behavioral problem or conflict in class, it is absolutely not appropriate to flip the classroom. Your students, while responsible for their own learning, are not responsible for disciplining other students.

Sometimes you may be able to flip classrooms with other teachers. Consider a class whereby you and a colleague are teaching the same subject, or one group has already had the subject. You can combine the two classes or flip so that one class has the other teacher. Let's say that you both are or have taught a class on cosmetic dentistry. Having students in the same class will allow them to discuss what they learned, and perhaps even discover some things they have not learned. Having the teachers flip will render the same result. Be on notice: this is not the time for students to complain their teachers didn't go over that material, but rather that they discovered some new information. Once again clear instructions must be present so that there is continuity between the two classes. This technique works exceptionally well with a skills-based lab, whereby more senior students can show their counterparts how to perform a skill they have already mastered. This will give the senior students a sense of confidence and pride as well as confirm they really know the material. Faculty should be on hand in case there is a question or if a technique is presented that does not follow the prescribed outline. Students often appreciate the opportunity to show off their knowledge, and this is a chance to do just that, while they also bond with peers.

Fear of Failure

We have reviewed a great deal of fun learning opportunities for you to use in the classroom. However, there may be times either you or your students hesitate for fear of failure. You may think, "I'm not good at that" or "I don't think I can pull this off," or even "The students will make fun of me." While you may not know how to, and may even stumble the first few times, you must venture into the unknown in order to grow. This is true for you as well as your students; the moment learning becomes familiar it can become stagnant. Choose just a few to start with and move slowly … perhaps even repeating it until you are sure it is not for you, or until it becomes part of your toolbox. And if you don't excel at one game, don't worry; even those who win "Teacher of the Year" aren't experts in everything.

In dealing with the fear of failure, some of the following exercises will help you realize where these fears are coming from. Being a teacher often means putting yourself on a stage for all to see; this can be quite scary and yet very humbling. It can also pull things out of you that you did not know you possessed, until you gave them the chance (who knew you were an artist?). Everyone has talents, and everyone has areas they need to improve on. As we continue to mature and grow into ourselves as human beings, we will discover more about ourselves that we will use in our profession. Have patience, believe you can, and be kind to yourself. Just as with your class, teaching needs to be fun while you are learning. Though often referred to as one of the hardest professions to work in, teaching can also be the most rewarding when you and your class are enjoying the process of learning.

Journal: Self-reflection

1 *Creating enticement*

a. As you reflect on that "education" buffet, what items would be most enticing to you if you were the student?

b. What would you be sure to include on your buffet if you were the "chef" for your students?

c. What other resources will you need to create the enticements needed to engage your students?

2 *MIT*

Let's revisit the various intelligences. In looking at your course and your students' learning styles, list four environments you will create which will engage students from at least three or more learning styles. Example: when using journaling you are tapping into their existential, intrapersonal, and verbal strengths. Outdoor activities encompass naturalistic, interpersonal, and intrapersonal strengths.

3 Create an account in each of the following sites: Quizlet, Poll Everywhere, and Kahoot! Write down your username and password (PW). Then create at least five items per the following instructions:

a. Quizlet: https://quizlet.com/sign-up
   Username:
   PW:
   Create five cards with definitions for your course. Write out the cards you have created here:

b. Poll Everywhere: https://www.polleverywhere.com
   Username:
   PW:
   Create five questions to poll to your students. Write your questions here:

c. Kahoot!: https://create.kahoot.it/register
   Username:
   PW:
   Create five questions with answers for your course. Write out the questions and answers you have created here:

4 *Jeopardy* (there are several websites you can use, one option is https://www.playfactile.com/)
Username:
PW:
You don't have to create an entire game, but at least two to three questions per category for at least two to three categories. The purpose of this is to try your hand with creating an engaging activity using technology. Write down the categories and a synopsis of the game here (as well as where you saved it):

5 *Other realities*

a. How do you feel about the use of VR and AR?

b. Have you had an opportunity to use, practice, or purchase these different realities? In the workforce? In education? Do you have any thoughts about how they might work in the class you are teaching?

c. If you could design a "futuristic" classroom using AR, VR, or other technology, how would it look?

6 Answer these questions on scale of 1 (not true) to 5 (absolutely!).
a. I feel comfortable using technology (in general): 1 2 3 4 5
b. I was comfortable using technology in the classroom (before this exercise): 1 2 3 4 5
c. I feel more comfortable using technology in the classroom (after this exercise): 1 2 3 4 5
d. I am confident students will enjoy this activity I created: 1 2 3 4 5
e. I am confident students will learn from this activity I created: 1 2 3 4 5

7 More games mean more engagement. Choose from the games mentioned in this book or other games you enjoy. Write down at least five that you will use in your class, as well as the tools or toys needed to carry them out (buzzers, music, etc.):

8 How will you use discussion or debates in your class? What topics might lend themselves to this form of engagement? List at least three topics you will use—state whether it would be a small group discussion, large group discussion, or a debate:

9 The sharing of personal experience is a great way to share on a topic you have already taught and need validation on, or simply wish to share another perspective on. What topics in your course would you use this form of engagement in? What resource(s) do you have to share (note: it does not have to be an outside speaker, but it needs to from the personal experience perspective):

10 Flipping the classroom sounds easy but does take some practice and preparation. How would you use this tactic? What activities could be instrumental in allowing the students to lead the learning in your class? List at least two situations where you would flip the classroom:

11 *Fear of failure*

a. What are some of your concerns, fears, or apprehensions on using or creating technology in the classroom?

b. Robert Schuller asks "What would you do if you knew you could not fail?" As a teacher, what would you do in the classroom if you knew you would not fail at it?

c. How do these concerns, fears, or apprehensions fit in with your ability to present your technology-based games to students?

____

____

____

____

____

____

____

____

d. What do you need to overcome these concerns, fears, or apprehensions?

____

____

____

____

____

____

____

____

12 Being your best means being the best that you can be. While it seems like a simple statement, it is often difficult to remember you are not always going to be engaging, fun, entertaining, and full of energy with new ideas. There will be days where you will need to get though some difficult material in a short amount of time, or perhaps you are not up to an invigorating discussion. Self-care is important but so is self-acceptance. Perhaps today—the best that you can do is be yourself. What does that mean to you?

____

____

____

____

____

____

____

____

It is the supreme art of the teacher
to awaken joy in creative expression
and knowledge
Albert Einstein

Chapter 5

Critical Thinking and Judgment

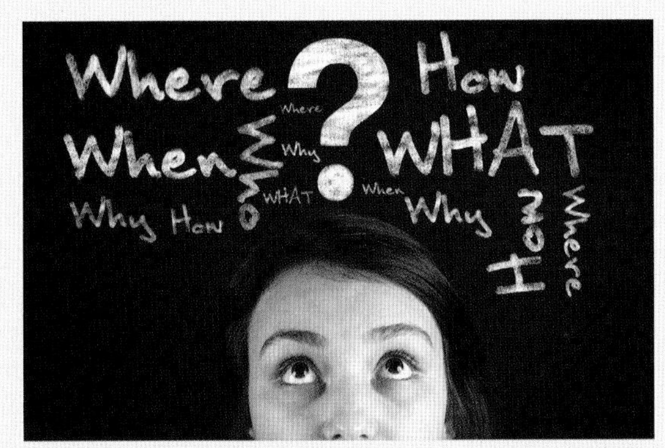

(turk_stock_photographer/iStock.)

What is critical thinking? Although there are several definitions, they all stem from how we draw our conclusions. As faculty and as students, we pull from a variety of resources, deductive and inductive reasoning, and draw from our own perspectives to analyze, then come up with a judgment, decision, or conclusion. To use critical thinking skills, we often must think outside the box, or outside of our own preconceived ideas or viewpoints in order to capture more unbiased perspectives. In order to do this effectively, there are several skills one must hone to be successful. However, the great thing about critical thinking is that there are no wrong answers (usually)—which is a nice stroke for fragile egos or those who are unsure of themselves. Faculty and students feel more relieved and are more eager to share their *angle* when they can do so freely and without judgment. It is important to note the distinction between judging others as right or wrong, versus creating one's own judgment (viewpoint, perspective, perception) based on the facts and opinions presented. Our review of these terms will eliminate the tendency to judge others, as this creates a wider gap on biases and does not achieve optimum learning. In critical thinking, one's own judgment is accepted, as we all have our own opinions. An important aspect in education is to be open to seeing things differently and welcoming all perspectives and opinions.

Critical thinking skills are used in every industry and are much sought after when employers are looking for the best candidate. Those who possess strong critical thinking skills can prioritize better, are often effective with time management, and know what is relevant and what is not when solving problems or conflict. For this reason, regardless of what class you are teaching, critical thinking will (or should) become a very important part of the class as well as in your preparation. This higher order thinking requires that students think outside of their comfort zone and rely on multiple angles and perspectives to draw conclusions. Though some textbooks may include critical thinking activities, others may not; incorporating critical thinking activities may be an aspect of the course you will have to introduce. While not difficult, it can take some time for the novice instructor to add these activities to their toolbox and be comfortable with these concepts. This chapter will guide you in how to best discover and hone these skills so you can use this technique to better guide students in their learning.

You Don't Know What You Don't Know

As comical as this statement is, we often forget that we don't know what to ask if we have no knowledge of the material nor any frame of reference. Consider a student who has never been to college. After you pull out your syllabus and share expectations, as well as the rubric for the final project, you may ask if anyone has any questions. The student who has no idea what a syllabus or rubric is won't even know what questions to ask. When reviewing assignments, syllabi, or even a task you feel is fairly simple or straightforward, be careful that you don't assume. This is where your own critical thinking comes into play. You want to start slowly and allow an opportunity to ask if everyone understands what these terms mean and what these tools are used for. If most of the class is familiar, but some are unsure, allow a peer mentor to those who may still be unclear. You may even choose to allow the peer mentor to spend some time with a small group after class. You may even challenge students' understanding by asking a few questions to confirm they understand, such as if the syllabus is a contract, and if so, what that implies.

The same concept is true when discussing most terms; you must ensure students have the same reference point. This is where critical thinking plays an active part, allowing various viewpoints and perspectives to come into play so that a greater understanding is formed. Often students don't realize that what may seem like common sense to one person has absolutely no reference point for another. Many words in the English language have multiple meanings or are polysemantic. Consider the words "bark," "lap," "current," and "pool"—each of these terms has more than one meaning. This is one reason why the English language is often hard to master for English as a Second Language (ESL) learners, as it can be quite confusing to know when to use each word in its proper context and appropriate definition. Many times, ESL learners get frustrated, or even embarrassed if they use the correct term in an incorrect context. However, it becomes more acceptable and even fun if the class looks at common terms and realizes the various contexts. The importance of understanding terms and the proper definition becomes even more important during a test. If a student does not know what a word means, it can make the difference in understanding what the question is (and thus the correct answer).

Although it can be difficult to ascertain what students don't know, it can be a point of reference for a student's engagement. Consider a game for students in small groups—they are given 10 common terms but must come up with various definitions. These terms may be part of your course or may be simple ones that have little reference to your class (as with the earlier examples). While it may not seem that this game correlates to your course, it does show relationships with words and perspectives, and how there can always be more than one "right answer." It also allows those who struggle with English (as ESL or in general with grammar) to freely ask for help, and to see how the terms make a difference when answering questions.

Why Is It Critical?

In Chapter 1 we reviewed learning theories and touched on cognition. Critical thinking takes cognition, or the inner workings of the brain, and supersizes the process; this is called metacognition, or thinking about how we think. When we can ask questions about what we see, hear, touch, and have learned, and go deeper into the thought process, we begin to realize our initial learning was superficial. As we delve further into the topic, concept, or process, our brains can encompass more information and piece together more complex and abstract information. This is what can separate college students from others, as they begin to ask more questions, challenge the answers, and create various layers of understanding versus accepting information "as is." Critical thinking uses various forms of reasoning, question and analysis, and probes the material being covered further; it is used in all subjects and can be a great way to instill wonder and discovery for student engagement.

Deductive and Inductive Reasoning

When it comes to reasoning, there is both deductive and inductive reasoning. Within each type of reasoning there are other terms and steps, such as inference, hypothesis, and conclusions. Although we will briefly cover each, it should be used as a backdrop in understanding critical thinking and how we gather information to come up with an answer. As we come up with our answers, we must realize that it is not the only answer, as nothing is ever proven in science. For starters, let's review the general concept of the scientific method. In the scientific method, the idea is to come up with a question or a problem, collect information regarding the issue, design a hypothesis or guess what the reason is, try it out, and determine if that intervention worked. If it is, we draw our conclusion based on our inferences or suggestions from our trial. If not, we repeat the step of trying it out.

An extremely simplified version of this is when a 3-month-old infant cries.

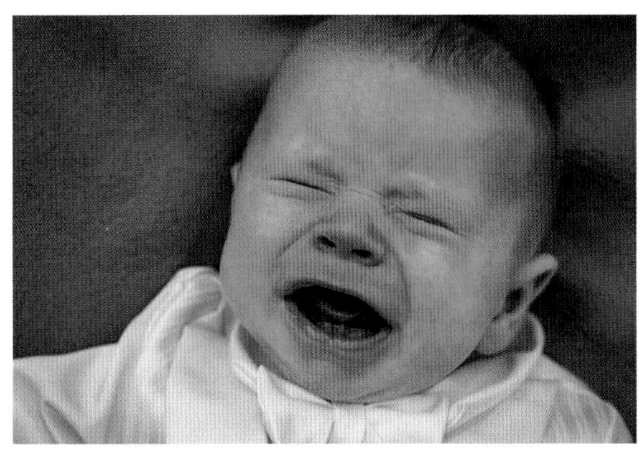

(NikonShutterman/iStock.)

- **Question/problem:** the infant is crying (why is he crying?).
- **Information:** tears are coming down the face of the infant and the infant is making a loud noise. It has been more than 2 hours since the infant was fed. The infant usually eats every 2–4 hours.
- **Hypothesis:** the infant is hungry.
- **Intervention:** offer the infant appropriate nourishment: breast, breastmilk, formula.
- **Result/Analysis:** if the infant stops crying, we were correct—the infant was hungry. If not, we return to another hypothesis: he could need a diaper change or could be lonely. Instead of being hungry, the infant needs a diaper change. We repeat the intervention step: check the diaper—is it dry or does it need to be changed? If it is soiled, we change it. If it is dry, we go to the next hypothesis, the infant is lonely. We go to the next intervention and hold/rock/coo with the infant in an attempt to soothe the infant.

Each of these steps are continued until we reach a conclusion. In the absence of any obvious issue, such as trauma, illness, or other apparent infraction of the infant's peacefulness, we would expect a simple answer to the simple issue of an unhappy infant. However, any parent knows that getting an infant to stop crying is not always so easy, or straightforward.

With deductive reasoning, there is a syllogism, composed of a major premise and a minor premise, which leads us to our conclusion. The major premise is a general idea or statement, followed by a secondary idea or statement. A common example is "all men are mortal" (major premise). George is a man (minor premise); therefore George is mortal. Both the major and minor premise are true, so we expect the outcome to be true. This syllogism can be viewed (for the logical and mathematical learners) as: A (men) = B (mortal), and C (George) = A (man), so therefore C (George) = B (mortal). However, these are generalizations, which may not be true. Consider the DC character Superman. While indeed all men are mortal, Superman (C) is a man (A), but he is not mortal (B). Aside from the fact that this character is fictional, it does show that sometimes A = B and C = A but C ≠ B. This is where critical thinking comes in and stops the assumptive clause.

As deductive reasoning goes from the general to the specific, inductive reasoning does the exact opposite: it goes from specific to general. Consider this example: your infant has cried every night during this past week. It is nighttime; therefore, your infant will cry. Of course, this is an assumption, or inference, and may not be accurate. Perhaps tonight is unique for some reason and your infant does not cry; perhaps the other nights were unique, and your infant does not cry during the night at all anymore (most parents' dream!). Inductive reasoning uses fact from a single occurrence (he cried at night for 1 week) to propose additional occurrences will have the same outcome (he will always cry at night). The inference that your infant will cry simply because he did so last week during the night is an example of inductive reasoning.

Along with inductive reasoning there is also abductive reasoning, which takes the generalization a bit further. In abductive reasoning, not all pieces have to be true to begin with. Let's say you hear a noise (similar to your infant's cry) and you walk into the nursery to find your infant in his bassinet. Your infant is quiet but has wetness on the cheeks of his face. Your 4-year-old daughter is in the nursery playing and tossing around some toys. Your assumption is that your daughter threw a toy which hit your infant and made him cry. When you question your daughter, she claims her baby brother was not crying, and that she did not throw any toy at him. While some parents would start with the assumption their daughter is lying (or stretching the truth), there are several other possibilities. Perhaps your son (the infant) was not crying, or not while your daughter was in the room; perhaps he was laughing. You would have to review more of the facts in greater detail to ascertain additional clues and come up with a different conclusion. Perhaps you missed the spray bottle of water that your daughter was using to clean her toys, which could explain the wet cheeks, the laughter (not crying), and why your daughter was correct. Her baby brother was not crying, and she did not throw anything at him.

As stated earlier, you need to remember that there is no proof in science—only theories and laws. Every situation can have more than one premise, more than one answer, and more than one outcome. While many students argue that there are proven theories, it is often a fun activity to ask students to list them. While they want to shout out certain scientific terms such as gravity (law), relativity (theory), and origin of our universe (theory), they will be stumped to discover that none of these are proven. Indeed, there are arguments to each of these, based on perspective from the additional facts and evidence. Not that you want to go down that rabbit hole with students, but it does support your lecture that there is no proof in science, and we can all make our best guess based on various factors.

Correlation and Causation

As we are discussing reasoning it is important to note that some students will want to assume correlation, meaning that because we did "x," then "y" will occur. Much like the inductive reasoning, just because two things appear to have a relationship does not mean it is the cause. Just because it is night, it does not mean your infant will cry. Just because students failed their first test due to ineffective study habits doesn't mean they will fail the second test. There may be a good chance if the study habits and test taking strategies are ineffective it can render the same results, but it is not a guarantee. In order to ascertain other outcomes, you must ask many questions.

Perhaps your child is afraid of the night, or at night a great deal of noise occurs, or you must leave to go to work at night; any of these situations can cause your infant to cry. With the increase in these situations the likelihood is greater that he will cry—not always, but there is a higher probability. Again, correlation does not mean causation: the night is not the cause of his crying. Likewise, the student who only reads their book to study for a test may fail one test, but not necessarily all tests. Asking questions to determine what other factors are involved and influencing the outcome is important.

Socratic Teaching

To take critical thinking to a more philosophical level, we need to go to our Greek ancestors, approximately 2500 years ago. The philosophers Plato, Aristotle, and Socrates were very influential in "education," or the quest for knowledge; they introduced a unique perspective which considered answers from within, instead of relying on external facts. Socrates was the teacher of Plato, who later taught Aristotle; these three philosophers were pivotal in the foundation and formation of Western philosophy and ethics. Socrates believed we possess all answers (and actually had them before we were born); we can discover these answers from within our own self through diligence, persistence, and the right questioning. This is where the adage "know thyself" stems from; although it is not a direct quote from Socrates, it does embrace his sentiment. Socrates' life work was in prompting and questioning others to seek their answers. It was believed that Socrates never wrote down any of his work, but rather used this original form of student engagement to allow his pupils to gain knowledge; knowledge, he believed, they already had. This form of teaching (by using questions to allow students to arrive at their own answers) is referred to as the Socratic method of teaching. This method has been used in all forms of education, most prominently in higher education. Although some current scholars claim there is a formal way to utilize the Socratic method, less stringent approaches see any form of questioning as supporting the Socratic method.

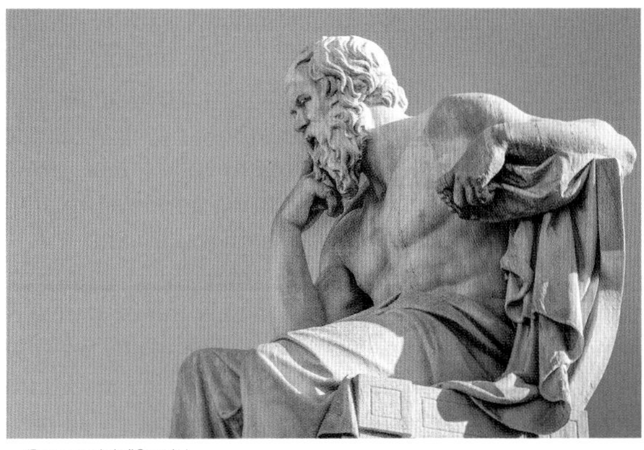

(Panasevich/iStock.)

Asking the Right Questions

The simplest form of Socratic teaching can come from the older child in the previous scenario. While you have assumed your infant is or was crying, your daughter is trying to discover why you are even in the room at all. A precocious child, she asks why you are here; you state because you heard a noise and thought it was your infant crying. She asks again, "but why are you here?" "Because," you respond, "if he is crying, I need to see what the matter is." Your daughter persists, but "why are you here?" Getting slightly annoyed at her questioning, you decide to amuse her one more time with a more definitive answer. "I'm the mommy, that's why!" Although there are a few 4-year-old children who would have the gumption to continue questioning why you were in the nursery, most might fear repercussion if they kept asking. However, should the questioning continue, the real reason you were in the nursey could stem from a deeper psychological issue, such as you are afraid you may not be meeting your infant's needs, or you fear your daughter may actually harm him, as she has been talking about how much she doesn't like her brother. Of course, it could also have nothing to do with any deep issue—you simply do not want to be inept at your parenting skills. While you may not be going for Mother of the Year, you do want to ensure your children are safe. To give your 4-year-old credit, why were you in the nursery at that particular time? Because you knew you had not checked on your infant in 2 hours and you thought (consciously or subconsciously) you heard him cry. You felt obligated to check on his safety, and a little guilty that you had so much quiet time. You assumed your daughter had hurt him (as she was tossing toys) and although you had no reason to doubt her safety or his, you began to explore the range of possibilities, starting with her as the guilty party.

Although we are not trying to compare 4-year-olds to college students, we can show a relationship in the art of questioning. Four-year-old children have an insatiable desire to seek the truth, or at least some version of it. They will continue to question until their own reality (truth) is at a point where they no longer need an answer. The final response of "I'm the mommy" was enough to quiet your daughter; although it didn't answer her question, she had no further need to ask another question. Her truth is that you are the mommy; her reality is you make the rules. Ergo, you are the mommy and you wanted to come into the room (for whatever reason you felt it necessary).

Why Ask Why?

Certain questions conjure up more than one answer, which is how the Socratic method truly is effective. If I ask you a closed-ended question, such as "what time is it?," the conversation has ended once you provide the time. Open-ended questions that ask "why?" and "how?" allow the responder to continue answering while the questioner guides the path. Let's use this example in a course on dental health. Suppose you are an instructor teaching this subject and have reviewed how important it is to brush your teeth, floss, and visit the dentist frequently for check-ups and routine cleanings. While your students take this information as normal expectations of good dental hygiene, you want them to know the rationale behind these practices. Why should you brush your teeth more than once a day? Why should you floss? Why should you see a dentist? Why should you even care about dental hygiene? Not to play devil's advocate (though you can), allow them to come up with an appropriate rationale for dental hygiene. You can add that they will most likely have some resistant patients who do not see the value in these practices (my teeth are going to all fall out anyway) and will have to explain why dental health is important. Questioning allows you to guide them in a deeper perspective; for example, the push for dental health is different for a 90-year-old man who has end stage liver disease than for a 12-year-old healthy adolescent.

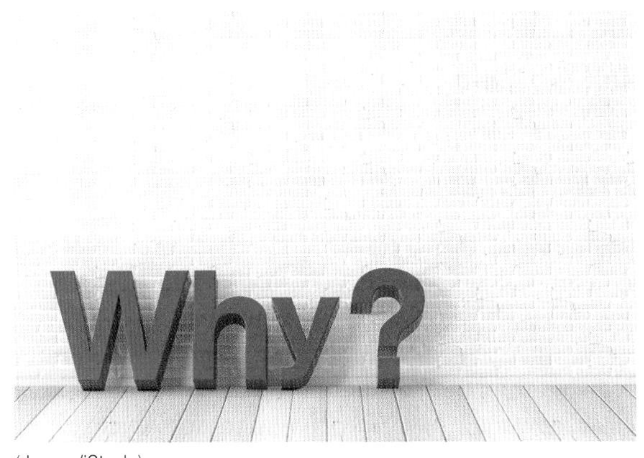

(doomu/iStock.)

Asking the "why" and "how" questions allows your students to come up with various right answers, their justifications, and to discover that many options are available. Let's consider another strategy with a class on nutrition. Many of the foods we eat nowadays are more prolific and disease resistant due to scientific influences of our food source. After reviewing the basics of nutrition, you begin to touch on the governmental impact of food production, such as genetically modified or genetically engineered foods. After explaining what these terms are, you may begin to ask such questions as: why would the government want to change a food? How would farmers do this? What could be some benefits to altering our food source? What are some concerns? Why are genetically modified organisms (GMOs) in foods considered "bad" for you? Are organic foods modified?

These conversations require some simple questioning at the conversational level but will also instill a deeper level of discussion as those with different points of view, such as the conspiracy theorists, land lovers, vegetarians, and the purely pragmatic students begin to argue their sides. It may even take some extra research to get their facts straight, but at first allow them to speak from the hip and share their viewpoints. The idea is not to split atoms on how food is genetically altered and whether it is safe, but why they feel it is or it isn't. Add to the discussion the question about how the government is supposed to feed an overpopulation of people they aren't ready for, and how we can compensate farmers without raising prices (particularly when discussing organic foods). The activity is to get students to think outside their box (the usual norm) and see various perspectives without solving the problem.

Tell Me More

As you can probably imagine, this sort of discussion can go on for hours with a chatty class but can also be ended quickly if everyone sees things from the same angle or has the same opinion. Therefore, your role is a pivotal one; as class facilitator (not necessarily the one with all the answers) you must challenge and guide each person's contribution. Moreover, you must regulate the pace so that those who have not voiced their viewpoint have an opening to do so, and those who control the floor can stop and listen to others. You will also want to interject more questions, to get them to think from an opposing side or to consider other people's values. This sort of discussion is particularly helpful in an area where concept mapping can occur. As you start with one idea and discuss it, it opens a Pandora's box of other ideas and can become the focal point of even more ideas. While some courses may not necessarily seem to lend themselves to the Socratic method, there is always a way to twist the class into asking "what if?"—even in a math class!

Concept Mapping

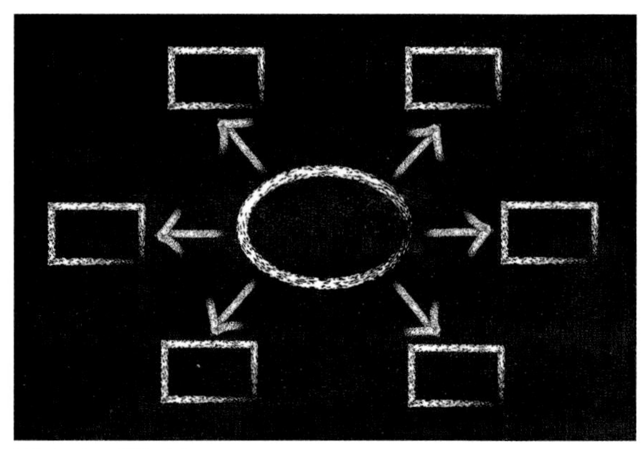

(akinbostanci/iStock.)

Concept mapping is used when discussing a subject that can have many implications, tangents, or associated topics. This mapping technique is used in many courses when there is a question, a problem, or a main point that can affect other outcomes. Let's use the example of the nutrition class and the discussion of modifying foods to feed the population. With food as the central concept, each tangent offers another aspect to the growth and production of food. For example, one circle or bubble (stemming from Food) includes the various governmental agencies (the US Food and Drug Administration [FDA], the US Environmental Protection Agency [EPA], and the US Department of Agriculture [USDA]) that regulate farming or food labeling; another circle includes the farmers themselves. From the circle with the governmental agencies, two other tangent lines are drawn—one circle for food safety (which the governmental agencies are responsible for) and one for the enhancement of food (which includes genetically modified foods and organic foods).

Stemming from the farmer are the many purchasers of foods (central suppliers), transportation of food, and so on. From each concept a line is drawn to another concept (or bubble); some tangents connect to more than one circle. As you can create this flow chart, start with one main concept then branch to each subconcept and sequential concepts that relate to the main topic. This requires some organization, but also creates a brainstorming session where students can offer multiple tangents and input based on a variety of subtopics. If other ideas creep up that may not be directly associated with this concept (such as unhealthy fast food), put it to the side. Either use this idea at another time or have a group of students build another map as a subsequent project.

Concept mapping has many benefits and requires little preparation. While it offers opportunity for impromptu discussions, a bit of prior planning is still needed. Remember, when the discussion lags, goes in a parallel direction, or students get stumped, you need to have provocative questions to promote critical thinking. One particular benefit is that this mapping can be done via software programs (search concept mapping apps) and on most Microsoft Office products (Word, PowerPoint [PPT], and Excel) as well as on a Mac computer. You can even draw it on a whiteboard, blackboard, or with sticky notes. If you have a beginning class and feel students may need some pre-set answers, you can hand out cue cards (index cards with an answer) or pre-made sticky notes and have students volunteer their answer when they feel it is an appropriate link to a concept. This will ensure student participation, as they have a correct answer for something—they may just need help connecting it to the right thought or defending why they feel a connection is there.

Student-Led Education

As we have covered in previous chapters, active learning or student-centered learning, whereby students are in charge of their own learning, requires more sophistication than passive learning. Critical thinking promotes this form of learning and encourages students to lead the discussion and be more engaged. Most classes will include an opportunity for critical thinking activities and thus allow the students to lead the learning. Not only is it a great way to engage students, it also lends itself to the idea of flipping the classroom (which was covered in Chapter 4). The more you, as the facilitator, can continue this energy the more the students will engage; soon, the energy becomes synergy and there is a positive spiral. When students are active in this process and gain more knowledge with more questions, they create a hunger within themselves. Often referred to as lifelong learners, they perpetuate more learning, as they are never satisfied with understanding one concept or answer. They constantly ask questions and learn from their quest. This form of learning was what Socrates deemed to be the crux of education, that we never know all the answers to any question, and constantly question all of the answers. As the answers are within us, we truly are trying to learn who we are and thus gain deeper awareness of how little we know about the world around us. This parallels Maslow's self-actualization, though Socrates might concede we never reach self-actualization.

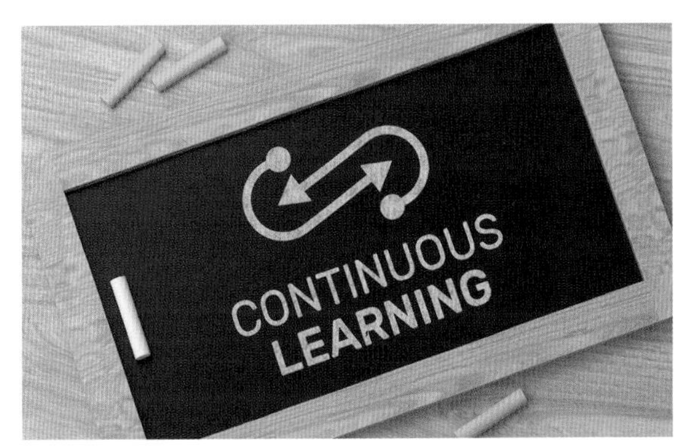

(GOCMEN/iStock.)

Your role in the lifelong learning process can be large or small, based on the student's own self-efficacy and trust. While one student may feel it is up to them to learn everything at their own pace, and your input is a negotiable contribution, other students may have more admiration for your expertise and take it with more than a grain of salt. Never take it personally if a student does not see your contribution to their education as significant; it could be they need to discover more on their own and through their own process of questioning various hypotheses. Again, you are the facilitator, not the answer guru. You can, in fact, promote more critical thinking when you put the questions back onto the students, as to why they need to pursue these hypotheses, and offer more controversial opinions and options for them to consider.

Compare/Contrast

There are various ways to use or promote critical thinking with class-based activities. One way is to ask students to compare and contrast two (seemingly) opposite ideas, concepts, or even people. Take for example, a class on leadership. When discussing great leaders, you may first start off with examples of characteristics such as being passionate about their cause, or compassionate and able to understand their followers. Once you have a list of great leaders and their characteristics, assign small groups to compare/contrast a few great leaders. Although they don't have to demonstrate completely opposite viewpoints, similar characteristics can be identified. Consider, for example, the assignment to compare and contrast two seemingly opposite fictitious figures: Darth Vader (from *Star Wars*) and Mufasa (from *Lion King*). Most students would wonder what these two have in common and wonder if you have lost your marbles. However, many great leaders demonstrate similar characteristics; for example, both Vader and Mufasa were extremely passionate leaders and were relentless in protecting their sons/kingdom/dynasty. They stopped at nothing to ensure that they could fulfill what they believed to be their purpose in life. They were instrumental and influential in their worlds and were both remembered for their passion; both were considered great leaders. Students, who may initially think these two have nothing in common, will have to use keen critical-thinking skills to come up with a list of similarities. For a livelier discussion (as if pairing these two leaders wouldn't be lively), you can also put various leaders' names in a hat and have students pick two names to compare/contrast. Though impromptu, it requires the use of critical-thinking skills as well as analytic thought processing. Students who have a bit more knowledge of these leaders can help lead the discussion, again focusing on even greater student engagement.

What's the Catch? "Four Out of Five Dentists Recommended"

When comparing and contrasting, we can get caught up in what is best and what supports the fact that it is the best. Whether discussing great leaders (and who is best), or food (is organic the best?), or even everyday products like toothpaste we go with what the rest of society thinks, instead of being our own critical thinkers. Social media has escalated this tainted view, as we get caught up in what the survey says, how many likes someone or something has, what the poll answers are, or what the leading research has shown. Any study, any research, survey, or poll can be skewed. This is not to negate these processes, or that research can and should be unbiased, but to elaborate on critical thinking. Everyone has seen their fair share of commercials (unless you are truly off the grid); most commercials for health products will have a tag line supporting the efficacy of the product. For example: certain toothpastes claim that four out of five dentists recommend their toothpaste for whiter, cleaner teeth, and their toothpaste is supported by the American Dental Association (ADA). Indeed, many toothpastes can whiten teeth, and all toothbrushes are designed to clean teeth. Any toothpaste that contains fluoride will most likely be supported by the ADA. And what about that fifth dentist who didn't support the toothpaste? All kidding aside, there is usually a specific (not an unbiased general) sampling of dentists who were pooled and used to promote a particular toothpaste. Most dentists recommend one toothpaste over another, and some may have even been paid for their support or promotion of the product. Without using critical thinking skills (which the toothpaste company is hoping you won't) you will assume their toothpaste is the best and purchase it.

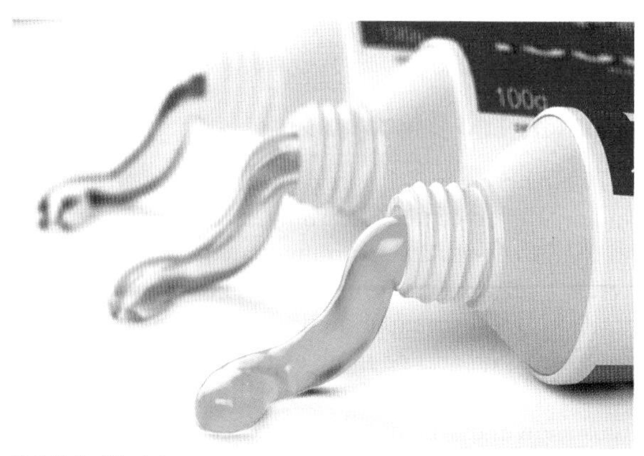

(Bet_Noire/iStock.)

Another example is the wide array of weight loss products. Weight loss products allege they have proven results (remember, nothing in science is proven) that their product will help you lose weight. These arguments can be a great way to kickstart the critical thinking process and dissect how such allegations can be made. Most weight loss products can *help* (operative word) a person lose weight, especially if they are motivated and change their eating habits and start exercising. This latter example begs the question: would the person have lost weight by changing their diet and exercising without the weight loss product? Allowing students to be devil's advocate or cynical in a scientific manner by dissecting these statements encourages their own self-learning and allows them to start the whole questioning process.

Despite the fun that can ensue with this sort of exercise, it is also important to remain professional. While toothpaste and weight loss products seem benign, other conversations may touch on a more delicate issue or hit closer to home for students (tobacco usage, for example). As these topics come up and you sense matters heating up, be aware of how all of the students are reacting and behaving. Students should never be encouraged to yell, use profanity, or become so rigid in their quest that they forget their manners. Politely disagreeing is a requirement of this or any exercise. Although some topics may be heated, and students may feel passionate about their questions, you, as facilitator, need to be the barometer. Allow breaks as needed, to let off steam or redirect the conversation; you may even have the class go out for a short walk to decrease any anxiety or to destress. Validating other's feeling, opinions, and perceptions can provide reassurance that everyone's viewpoint is acceptable and their perception is noted. Breaks also give you and the class a chance to regroup and return with a better awareness of the topic at hand, perhaps without as much emotional energy (if it was a controversial topic).

As the facilitator, you want to guide the conversation, the essence of comparing, contrasting, and arguments, in a specific direction. While the toothpaste example primes the discussion, direct the next topic to one that is important for your class. In our nutrition class, that weight loss product is a great segue to discussing eating disorders, such as anorexia, bulimia, and binge eating. As you enter these discussions, realize that at least one of your students may have been affected by this disorder—tread softly into the discussion but with a purpose. (This is why the cool down period is important, so that students can retain an open mind and have compassion when listening.) Maintaining sensitivity but also objectivity will allow you to review the main concepts and encourage others to share their experience or awareness of this disorder. Think of yourself as the train conductor: you are following a path to a destination, as the students enjoy the journey you reference various points of interest along the way. As their guide, you may not know everything, as you are part of the journey as well. With your guidance, you bring students to a deeper awareness and more knowledge about the subject material. Your guidance is not from happenstance; in Chapter 2 you planned this course on purpose with specific objectives in mind. Whether or not the students realize it, your path leads them through each step in their taxonomy of learning as they begin to master the subject at hand.

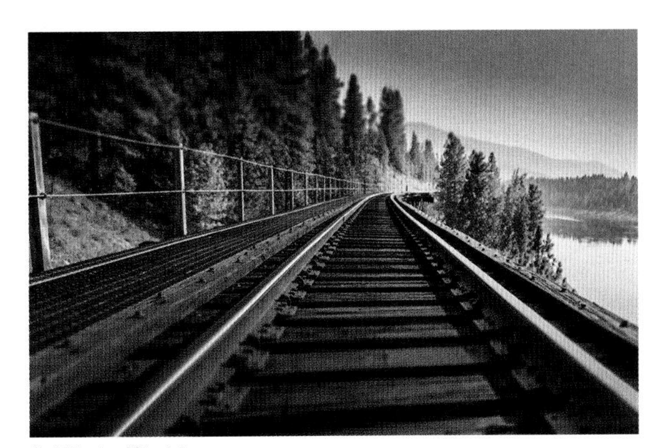

(keithbwinn/iStock.)

Bloom's Taxonomy

In Chapter 1 we reviewed Bloom's taxonomy and the various levels of learning. This taxonomy guides the faculty to direct that train through each level, as we pursue a higher order of thinking. Going through each level is not a race, but rather an opportunity to become more grounded in one aspect of learning before moving on. Your course may not necessarily be the highest level of material for the student's program (as each course is scaffolding to the next). However, each course can have its own higher order of learning. For example, in teaching a math class, your class may be a basic review course and may not go into advanced trigonometry or calculus, but you can still achieve all levels of the taxonomy within your own basic math course. Within each course there should be advancement of each level in Bloom's taxonomy. The six levels are listed below to give you some ideas of how to use this in your own class. At the end of this chapter, you will have a chance to list the exercises you wish to include that explore each level of Bloom's taxonomy. As always, you are welcome to make this a student engagement activity and ask them ways to remember materials, evaluate, or create. (For a visual reference of the pyramid refer to Chapter 1.)

REMEMBERING/KNOWLEDGE

This is the basic level and a starting place for all classes. Students will begin to use rudimentary skills to cover concepts in their initial few days of the course. As they begin to learn these fundamental concepts, you will check their knowledge base by asking them to recall what they have learned (or what they can recall from a prior course or prior education) and what is still fuzzy. Activities should be focused on the task or concept; for example, a few weeks into a basic anatomy class, ask students to list or name the major systems of the body. Have students describe each system's function and list the organs involved. Bring a blank diagram of the body and ask students to find where each organ should be or provide a model of the body and ask students to point to where the organ belongs. In this level of learning, students should be writing down material and repeating it. Though not always the best learning technique, this level does require some form of memorization and repetition. When students can demonstrate where the organs are located and which system they belong to, they have shown that they can remember the material. However, this does not necessarily imply they understand *why* the organ belongs to this system. Even animals can remember, but not necessarily understand.

UNDERSTAND

Once they can recall information, do they understand it? Can they explain it? At this level, it is important that you allow some form of discussion so that students can begin to process this information. Class activities should be focused on the students showing their understanding through interpersonal communication, such as small group presentations. Have students (individually or in small groups) describe the organ and its function and how it works within the system; how does it work with other systems? Can they predict outcomes or anticipate what would happen if the system failed or if there was something obstructing the system (such as a disease or disorder)? Their ability to recognize new information, such as a diseased organ, allows them to demonstrate knowledge of the basic concept (healthy organ) and the fact that something is different. Our previous reference to comparing and contrasting topics provided good activities that begin to show understanding.

APPLY

Once students believe they really do understand the information, how can they apply it to the real world or a hypothetical situation? If you cover the material on organs and systems and throw in a monkey wrench with a disease or dysfunction, what then? Can students continue to follow the pathway of the pancreas, for example, when it has damaged islets of Langerhans or no insulin being produced? While you are directing them to learning about type 1 diabetes, you need them to start their critical thinking wheels pointing toward the "what if's?" What if our pancreas does not produce insulin—what other systems would be involved? How would our diet be affected? While you cover these areas, you also bring in new information—the skill of checking glucose. After teaching students this skill, not only do you want to ensure that they can in return demonstrate the skill, you also want them to start piecing the puzzle together. Vignettes or short case studies (uncomplicated) can begin to allow students to solve the mystery, so to speak, and apply this learning to real life.

ANALYZE

The ability to analyze, dissect, or take apart a topic and re-create it shows a significant contribution to learning, as the students discover tools to determine what is right or wrong, appropriate and relevant, or doesn't belong. Activities which assimilate common ideas and differentiate them (on a deeper level than comparing and contrasting) can reveal their ability to analyze. This level of understanding is used in every class (including English and math), though it is more obvious in the health profession, criminal justice, and psychology courses. Consider a developmental psychology course where students can analyze a child's behavior through interviews, observations, and testing. They pull from each of the pieces of data to ascertain why the child acts out or has temper tantrums. They will be required to look at different angles (home, school, and social relationships) as well as the use of testing. They cannot simply recall their study of the brain or psyche or be able to apply it to a child; they must be able to pull pieces together to form an opinion, synopsis, and analyze various components. Activities that use puzzle solving skills, such as complex case studies, are best in this level.

EVALUATE

When the student is able to analyze, they can better differentiate what belongs, what doesn't, what is important, and what is not. They begin to calculate the value of each piece of data to determine its effectiveness or contribution to the concept. In the earlier example of the child acting out, the faculty member offers several pieces of data to create the backstory: the child is a first-born 8-year-old boy who was recently adopted. He is of Asian descent and has no other siblings. Even though he is a diabetic, he enjoys eating sweets; ice cream is his favorite. His father is very strict and often scolds him for his poor diet choices, as it affects his blood glucose levels. His mother, in an attempt to offset the father, offers him treats on the side. His (adoptive) parents are African American, and his mother is a stay-at-home mother. He lives in an affluent neighborhood which is in a country-like setting; many of the families do not have children but do have several pets. He likes to play with the neighborhood animals. Based on their analytical skills, students can decide what is important to note (remember, this is a developmental psychology class, not nutrition). While the child's interest in sweets is noted, it is not the primary factor in ascertaining why the child acts out. Asking students to rank each factor and note their importance allows them to ascertain the weight of each piece of information and what is missing. They are better able to choose what might affect this child's behavior and what could be in the periphery. While the diagnosis of diabetes may not rank high, the fact that there are no other children around to play with is of concern. Students should be able to recognize that this social isolation (if present) could contribute to the child's frustrations; it can also add to the fact that this child knows he is "different" (coupled with the disease process). When students evaluate this situation, they can also make recommendations or suggestions. They prioritize questions (are there other children to play with—perhaps scheduled play dates or sports activities? Are there cousins or other children in the family?). This level of learning also lends more to debates as students are required to justify and defend their position. While one group may feel the social isolation is contributing to the child's behavior, another group may feel it is the strict father and countering mother which is sending mixed signals to the child. Many of the activities we have reviewed that refer to the higher order of thinking are revealed in the students' abilities to evaluate.

CREATE

The highest order of thinking requires the students to create a whole new case, to compose a new material. They can use their imaginations to construct more ideas and investigate additional concepts to add to their own learning. In this example, students could fill in all the missing pieces and extrapolate on the need to have a session with the parents, child, and schoolteacher to review the underlying issues at hand. Though hypothetical, students can use their expertise to create a plan of action, complete with interventions and suggested follow-up questions, for all parties involved in this boy's care. They can surmise the impetus behind the behavior according to various theorists (Jung, Freud, Piaget), and show how each theorist would recommend proceeding.

A Faculty Member's Own Use of Bloom's Taxonomy

While all courses offer the opportunity to implement each step of Bloom's taxonomy, faculty also need to use this taxonomy for their own learning. Chances are, as a new teacher, you are (or were) at a point of simply remembering basic concepts. You will have to recall information from your own prior learning and gauge its effectiveness. You will take these concepts and apply them to your specific course or class. From there, you will analyze their effectiveness and determine how to augment prior ideas into better ones. You will continue to evaluate and create new lesson plans, continuing this cycle as you become engaged in the process of your own lifelong learning. It is no coincidence that this handbook is designed the same way: using the same steps of recall, understand, apply, analyze, evaluate, and create in each chapter, as well as the reflection activities. Within each chapter, and each topic within each chapter, there are more ideas from which to build on, which adds to your toolbox. As you go through your course, keep in mind that you are a student as well. Even though you are well versed in the subject matter, there are more ways to extrapolate the material and more effective ways to teach it to others.

Games That Promote Critical Thinking

Games, in general, promote critical thinking. Whether they are puzzles, interactive games, small group projects, or even video games (yes, there is a great purpose for video games), our brain is stimulated and we want more. And the more we play these games, the better our brain assimilates the information and accommodates the space for additional information. This can be easily illustrated with the example of a video game. Whether you are playing Pac-Man or a massively multiplayer online role-playing game (MMORPG), there is a strategy involved. In Pac-Man you'll want to eat the dots and blinking energizers—those red, blue, and yellow guys (don't forget the fruits); in MMORPGs you may want to take over another colony, annihilate the bad guys, and create your own country with a better army. Each game requires you to do multiple activities and get to the "next level" (even the arcade game Pinball does this). These activities invigorate the brain and get you thinking about thinking (metacognition) on how to get to that next level. It is very active (there is nothing passive about a video game!), engaging, and keeps you interested (no sleeping either). This is also why these games are so compelling, as they produce an enjoyment not found elsewhere. Of course, your classes may not be as addictive, but they can certainly fill a void in a student's lifelong learning process.

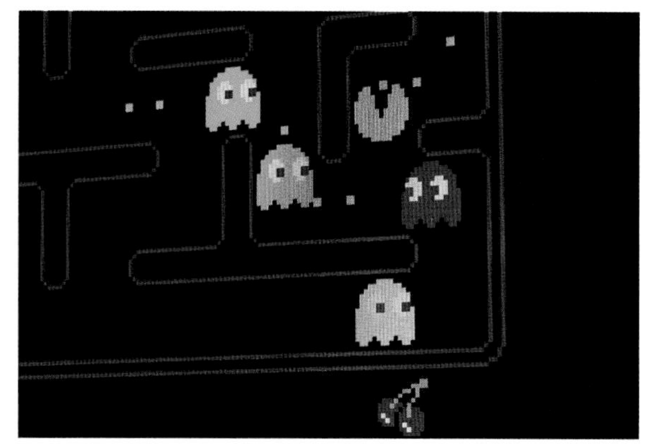

(ilbusca/iStock.)

In addition to video games there are card and board games that can be used as a critical thinking activity. *Apples to Apples*, *Cards Against Humanity*, and *Heads Up!* are popular critical thinking games that can allow players to connect abstract concepts not normally put together. While some of these games are more suited for social events (an adult party at home), you can draw off of their style and fashion them to be appropriate for the classroom.

Memory games are easy to re-create in the classroom and can be used for any situation. Although recall seems to be the most obvious level of learning, you can have students write a page on the subject but leave out specific (and important) words. These missing pieces become the framework to test their peers' knowledge. For example, in our class on anatomy, have students pair up: one as the creator, one as the doer; then have them switch. The creator makes a short "quiz" on their favorite system (or the one you just covered). They must have a variety of ten questions with labeling, fill in the blanks, and matching exercises on the system. Let's say the creator chooses the cardiac system—they would review the cardiac system and claim it has major parts that are necessary in order to function; some parts push blood one way, other parts push blood another way. After a brief overview of the cardiac system (leaving out specific terms/parts), the doer must then list the four chambers of the heart, the valves used, and the vessels. The doer must also review how the blood flows from one chamber into the other and to the lungs and back. To ensure the participants use all levels of Bloom's taxonomy, you ask the creator to include a short essay question, such as what symptoms would we see in the cardiac system if the respiratory system, or lungs, failed? While memory is involved, as the doer must recall these major anatomical components of the heart, you have also interjected the level of evaluation by asking that short essay question. In addition, the creator has performed the highest level of Bloom's taxonomy; not only must they create the memory game, they must know the answers and defend why the short answer is correct or wrong.

Trivia is the best use of critical thinking, whether used in jokes, common-sense scenarios, or seemingly unrelated facts. Take for instance the scenario of 12 members on a plane: three are Canadian, four are American, and five are Asian. The flight came from Japan and will go to New York, but first it will stop in Calgary, Canada. However, during the flight there is turbulence and the engine malfunctions. The plane ends up crashing along the US–Canadian border and there is controversy as to what to do with the passengers, as some are severely injured. While there is a hospital nearby, there is the reality that the emergency crew will not be able to reach the scene in time to offer the necessary medical interventions. You ask your students: "Where should we bury the survivors?" The answer, of course, is that we don't bury survivors. However, some students may not catch on as quickly and begin to ask some interesting questions. Another "common-sense" scenario is to ask students to consider a windup clock; you must get up at 0900 but you are very tired. You set the alarm (for 9 a.m.) but go to bed at 2030 (8:30 p.m.). How much sleep did you get? While students want to bring out their calculators and derive a math question to come up with their answer of 12.5 hours, they are stumped when you say 30 minutes. Most wind-up clocks do not differentiate between a.m. and p.m.; from 8:30 to 9:00 you slept and then the alarm woke you up 30 minutes later.

There are many trivia questions which can be created for any class. The popular board game *Trivial Pursuit* has various versions and different categories in each. While the category may not be in direct alignment with your course, it can initiate conversations that are. For fun, you ask your students (in anatomy or nutrition class): "What is the world's most densely populated island (hint: it's not Oahu)?" (As of this writing, it is Santa Cruz del Islote in Colombia, near Bolivar.) While this piece of trivia might win you a round on *Jeopardy*, what does it have to do with anatomy or nutrition? Using this example to initiate a conversation that compares this tiny man-made island to the islet of Langerhans gives a better appreciation for the beta cells used to produce insulin. In fact, when considering this island is only about three acres wide and has slightly over 1200 people, you can elaborate on the importance of efficiency, the need to rely on bigger spaces (aka organs) to help production, and what would happen if there were a disaster (disease). While this comparison may seem like a stretch—it can get you and your students on a very engaging discussion using a variety of skills and knowledge. If nothing else, at least you drew the class in with something that seemed trivial and kept their attention focused on something that is perhaps more important.

Small Group Projects

As mentioned, critical thinking is done in both intrapersonal activities (solo) and interpersonal (social) activities. Small group projects allow various learning styles to work together to feed off one another's strengths and improve on weaker areas. Pairing students in activities can be a great use of this strategy as you utilize various learning styles and knowledge background to blend students' understanding into a broader experience. Previous strategies that were discussed included think/pair/share and flipping the classroom. These activities promote critical thinking as students continue to lead the quest for more knowledge and recap what they have learned. It is important that you respect individuality and creativity. A rubric should be clear when students lead presentations, but also afford them an opportunity to speak freely without judgment.

Different Perspectives

When pairing students in small groups, especially to maximize Bloom's taxonomy and the use of critical thinking skills, you will need to draw on their differences. Divide groups based on a variety of characteristics and ensure each group has different genders, ages, culture or ethnicity, and possibly even religion (if appropriate). This blend will ensure that diverse perspectives are included and that students have more than one representation of any category. By blending the groups, the outlook is less controlled as their differences will offset their similarities. You can monitor these activities but also control them with role playing. Assign behaviors to students and have them participate according to that role. When discussing cardiac care and nutrition, have one student be the physician, one be the dietician, one be the patient, and one be the patient's significant other. While the physician wants to order cardiac medicines to lower the patient's blood pressure, the dietician feels the diet is a more conservative approach as the patient enjoys a heavily salted diet, doesn't exercise, and smokes. The student playing the significant other role is defiant about the patient not changing his lifestyle. He argues about every diet, every medication, and says there is no need for him to change his ways. In fact, as the patient is over 50, he should be allowed to live his remaining years the way he wants.

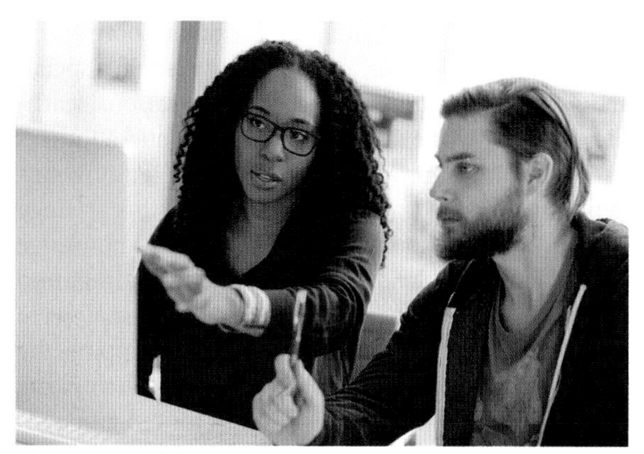

(FangXiaNuo/iStock.)

Diversity offers different perspectives, but it also forces each participant to use their own critical thinking skills. When students can take on a role, and the behavior associated with it, they can get a better or more accurate perspective and ask *different* questions. If the mentioned scenario was presented to the class, students may come up with some questions about the patient's right to choose. However, as the patient's significant other (whether an intimate partner, parent, son, or daughter) argues that the patient has the right to live his life the way he wants, more objectivity may ensue from the audience (other students). They may be better able to gain compassion and relate to the scenario as a spouse, parent, child, or friend. "If this were my significant other, I would also be an advocate to let them live their life as they want," or "as an advocate for good health, I would want my loved one to live as long as possible, and would substitute some of their bad habits for good ones so that I can enjoy being with them longer." Using role play with critical thinking activities can maximize your impact on understanding different perspectives. However, be cautioned, as it can also raise concerns and judgments.

Judgments

Critical thinking requires us to look at situations from various angles, without judgment. However, it is human nature to judge. How then do you, as the faculty member and the facilitator, prevent others from judging? The easy answer is you can't. You can't control your students' thought processes or how they feel. You cannot open their minds or their hearts and see where their responses are coming from, nor can you outwardly change them. You cannot control how they perceive information or how they react. You can, however, ensure there is a neutral ground as much as possible. You can be open minded yourself, listening to even the most controversial ideas and most outlandish viewpoints, without judgments. Though it may not seem like it makes a difference, it models professional behavior. It gives students a safe place to share, to know that while they may judge others, they will not be judged. This is crucial to gain the trust we mentioned earlier; the more they trust you, they more students will share who they are. As you recall from Chapter 3, your class may be the only safe place they have to share.

Journal: Self-reflection

1. What don't you know (yet)? Considering the topics we have covered, there may be a few that you are more unfamiliar with. Don't be embarrassed, write them down so that you have a point of reference for later. Write down at least five areas you want to learn more about.

2. In reviewing the concepts of deductive, inductive, and abductive reasoning, think about your course. What issues are prevalent in your industry? What problems could arise within your subject matter—such as hypertension (when teaching cardiac health) or dental caries (when teaching dental hygiene). Come up with at least six problems based on your subject matter for which students could apply the scientific method. You won't write out each step right now, as you will need to review this as part of your course planning. For now, simply identify those six problems.

3. Considering your class, anticipate at least two problems that can arise while conducting the activities you planned (students are not engaged, students get loud, boisterous, and argue, students leave class). Using the scientific method, go through a brief step-by-step contingency plan for the what if:
First problem:

a. Observations or other information to substantiate this is a problem:

b. Your hypothesis (why there is this problem):

c. Intervention (what you plan on doing to decrease or eliminate this problem):

d. What result you expect from this intervention:

e. *If* this intervention doesn't work, next steps:

Second problem:

a. Observations or other information to substantiate this is a problem:

b. Your hypothesis (why there is this problem):

c. Intervention (what you plan on doing to decrease or eliminate this problem):

d. What result you expect from this intervention:

e. *If* this intervention doesn't work, next steps:

4 Correlation versus causation is a common error when students look at problem-solving activities. It is easy to assume that "A" is a result of "B"; however, after reviewing this concept you know that is not the case. Identify at least three topics/subject areas within your course whereby you will have students look at how the causation is/is not a result of the correlation. Example: heart disease is linked to obesity, but not every person with a heart condition is obese; not every obese person has a heart disease.

5 Not everyone is comfortable with the methods used in Socratic teaching.

a. What is your comfort level? Select from the range of 1 = a lot of anxiety about this style to 10 = very comfortable with this method of teaching. If you have not had the chance to use this method, what do you anticipate your comfort level to be?

b. What are some methods you will use that support this style of teaching, based on your comfort level?

c. How can you increase your comfort level with Socratic teaching? Whom do you have to go to for help or what other resources can you draw from?

6 We covered the idea of using a Concept Map. Consider one topic within your course where this style of teaching would be appropriate. Draw your concept map below; be sure to use at least three additional circles in addition to the main one and at least two offshoots for each.

7 Compare and contrast activities require some forethought. Think of a topic in your class where you can use this method. What would you have the students compare/contrast?

8 Consider a major topic in your course where you will use each level of Bloom's taxonomy. Using the taxonomy, outline each level and the activity you will create (or have students create) to reach this level:

a. Recall:

b. Understand:

c. Apply:

d. Analyze:

e. Evaluate:

f. Create:

9 Playing games—as mentioned we want to encourage games to promote critical thinking skills. In addition to the games you already identified in Chapter 4, list at least three additional games that will promote critical thinking skills in your class:

10 Diversity is important for great critical thinking. How will you deflect or deter judgments? How will you create an atmosphere that encourages diversity?

What are some pitfalls that you need to be cautious of when planning these activities?

11 What concerns do you have about using critical thinking in your class?

I know that I am intelligent, because
I know that I know nothing
Socrates

Chapter 6

Best Practice for Effective Instruction

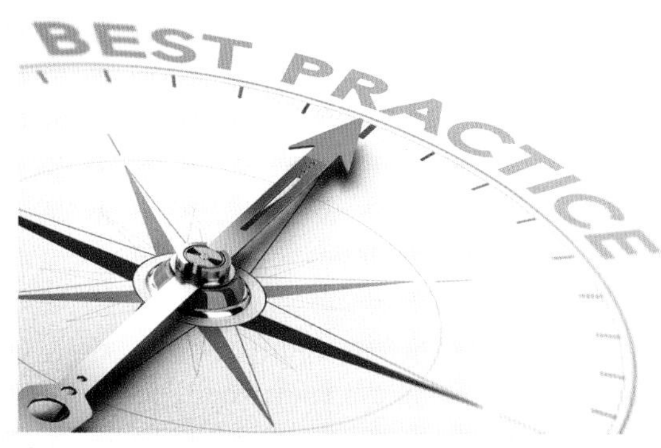

(Olivier Le Moal/iStock.)

Now that we have had a chance to review the basics, we will get into more of the details. We will go back over the first five chapters with respect to best practices and point out what is most effective (according to some general rules). Before we do that, let's dissect these terms: best, practice, effective, instruction. As you have (hopefully) learned, most learning is based on perspective. So, what is your perspective? While you will have an opportunity to reveal some interpretations and perspectives at the end of this chapter during the reflection aspect and provide some personal answers to this question, we will do an overview of each of these terms.

Consider, for example, something you may not necessarily be good at, but you enjoy: singing, sewing, painting, dancing, sports, cake decorating, whatever it is. You enjoy this activity, whether you do it well or simply in the privacy of your own space. If you are not great at this activity, you may not perform it publicly or do it for others, but when no one is looking, you go full force and give 100% to this activity. You'd love to be an expert at this thing, but the truth is, you do it for fun. These activities are great for stress relief and connect us with our inner creative being (perhaps you call it your inner child). These activities are important to guide us with our strengths and areas where we want to improve. And believe it or not, these activities can help you be a better teacher.

However, teaching is not just for fun; you have lives at your disposal, and these lives matter. While you may have fun while teaching, it is not a spectator sport, a weekend game, or even a hobby. This means you must take it to heart at some level, use your mind at another level, and take it with a grain of salt at another level. While it is your job to be a teacher, that is what you are hired to do, most institutions also ask that you continuously improve your teaching approach. No doubt you are held to some standards and will be reviewed for your ability to reach these standards. These evaluations (whether based on performance, merit, or actual observations) are for Human Resources (HR) and are important. However, they may not evaluate how *effective* you are as a teacher. Understanding these terms according to your own interpretation and according to your industry is paramount in becoming a better, or more effective, teacher.

So back to these terms. Everyone has a unique definition of these terms; do not feel there is a right answer, or that one expectation will fit all faculty. Just as we have stated with students—everyone has their own perspective. Your perspective, your expectations of yourself (and of the teaching industry), is important to review. When it comes to judging whether you are using best practices and are effective in your own instruction will vastly depend on your internal barometer and judgment of your own self. It also will depend on how you, personally, define these terms and their value to your teaching style.

Best

Too many times we feel that we must be the best, number one (#1), with little room for anything else. Sayings such as "no one can do it better," we are the "cream of the crop," "top of the heap," and "among the elite" make us feel that anything less is second best. We want to receive those affirmations, accolades, and confirmations that we are good, smart, competent, and capable. We think we must strive for perfection, even if we never achieve it. We don't often recognize progress, as we keep our eye on the goal: to be perfect. The flip side is, of course, that we will never reach perfection, never be good enough, never be #1. We are striving to simply survive, be accepted, and know that we have done our best in the end. Stepping outside yourself and looking at what "best" is can be a good first step. Who says this practice is the best? How do we determine what is the best? What does "best" mean with practice if we never reach perfection? These are internal questions that often cause the new faculty to hesitate in thinking or believing they can ever be the best. However, performing best practices really has nothing to do with you, per se. It has to do with how your teaching met the needs of the students. It has to do with what measure you employed to ensure students had the opportunity to learn. And it has everything to do with your students. What is good, best, or effective for your students may not work for another group of students. As we have reiterated, knowing your audience and what their needs are is crucial in understanding what is best, that is, what is working in instruction so that these students learn.

Best practices need to rely on current practices. What is effective today may not be effective 5 years from now, or even with the next class. Best practices are the ones that are most relevant and most relative to your students, today. Best practices may be something from the past that has been updated, not outdated. While this may seem obvious, we often get so focused on our planning we forget to update and refresh our plan. Your students are the indicators as to what is best. Best does not mean most enjoyable, but rather what is the most direct or successful path that leads them to the goal.

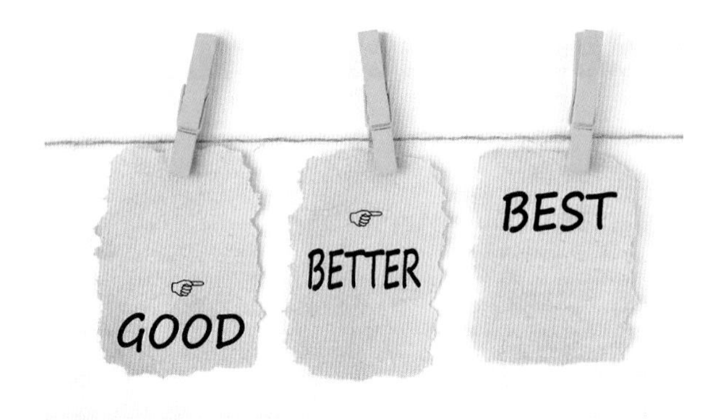

(ogichobanov/iStock.)

Practices

Practice implies you are not done, as you are still practicing. So, what are you striving for? What are you attempting to ascertain? As you teach, what do you want in return? How will you know when you get it? What will it look like? As stated earlier, you are not perfect, and neither will your teaching be. You will have great days and not so great days, and some days in between. Although we hope to have more great days than not so great days, we are constantly a work in progress. Education and learning are fluid, not static. They evolve, change, and are continuously being molded and shaped based on myriad other factors; in its own world, education is trying to keep up with an industry that is ever changing. Whatever subject you are teaching, that industry is also evolving, changing, and is not static. So how can you practice in an ever-changing merry-go-round? Before you get too dizzy, keep in mind that there are millions of other teachers, doing the same thing. As teachers, we are in our world of discovering how to help our students reach their goals. That's what practice is all about—we try it out, see if it works for this student, and try something different if it doesn't. Because these industries are constantly evolving, we must keep up with the evolution and be willing to make changes. Some may be a slight tweak; others may be a bigger overhaul. To continue to practice new things and be open to new ideas means we are practicing to be better than before.

Effective

One of the most important words in this chapter title is "effective." What does this word mean to you? How will you know if your class or course is "effective"? Often, we get confused with what went well versus what is effective. One of the easiest ways to determine whether the class went well on any particular day is to ask your students directly. However, effective does not necessarily mean that it was a fun class. Some peripheral items may also determine whether your class was effective: did you start and end on time? Did you finish your assignment, the class you planned? It all starts with what the goal was for that day, the class, or the overall course. Once again, we must begin with the end in mind.

Effectiveness means that the goal or objective was met. Whether it is that indeed you did start and end on time (a small accomplishment which you have not had a chance to do in 8 weeks), all of your students passed their test (first time ever), or you finally got everyone to openly discuss a topic, you reached a goal. In goal setting, remember to make your goals very specific; vague goals do not allow for any evaluation. Your goals must be measurable; the person who attempts to judge whether you met your goals (whether yourself or someone else) must have an objective means to do so. Are your goals attainable? Asking everyone to enjoy a class, for example, is not attainable for every class. You must set realistic goals for yourself. Your goals must be relevant to what you are doing; they need to match up with the activity at hand. Finally, there must a realistic time frame in which you anticipate the goal(s) being met. These steps can easily be illustrated with this example of a person who wants to lose weight.

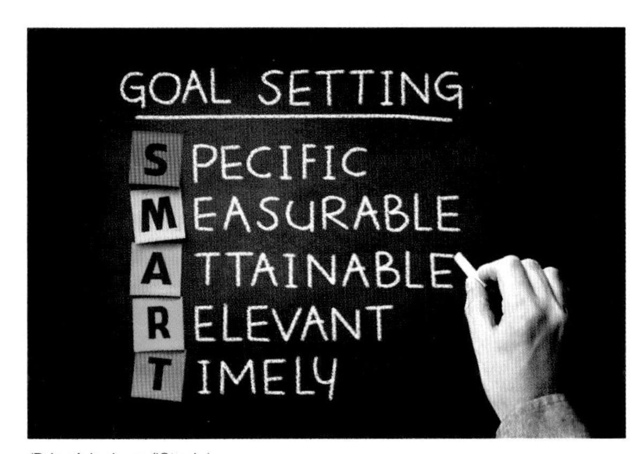

(BrianAJackson/iStock.)

Scenario: A 20-year-old Asian woman, Mia, feels that she is overweight and wants to lose weight. She wants to lose 30 pounds (lbs.) in 4 weeks. She currently weighs 120 lbs. and stands 5'8". Her friend, Emily, says she will join in this quest and also wants to lose 30 lbs. However, Emily feels that 4 weeks is too rigorous; she would like to lose the weight within 8 weeks. Emily stands 5'6" and weighs 180 lbs. Both women tend to eat junk food and have not been exercising. They are committed to eating less refined sugars and including more fresh fruits, vegetables, and lower fat foods in their diet. While not following a specific diet or exercise plan, they will walk at least 2 miles a day and increase it to 5 miles each weekend day. They have a reliable scale to weigh themselves every week. While this seems like a great plan, let's dissect whether or not it is SMART (specific, measurable, attainable, relevant, timely).

Specific: Mia's and Emily's goal is somewhat specific: to lose 30 lbs. This is different from a person saying they simply want to lose weight—they have a number in mind and know their starting point (in pounds). However, it does not account for other factors such as simply losing water weight or gaining muscle (which can occur when adding exercise). More specific factors could include reducing a dress/pant size or reducing measurements around "fatty" areas (arms, hips, thighs, etc.).

Measurable: Being that they have a reliable scale, they can do a weigh in; however, they must also be careful to weigh in each week at the same time. Other measurements should be included to ensure they are not simply trading fat for muscle. Measurements on waist, hips, buttocks, and arms can offer more accurate data and follow a more specific goal.

Attainable: In Mia's case, while this goal may be attainable, it is very restrictive as her body mass index (BMI) classifies her as underweight. There may be serious side effects to losing such an amount of weight, especially in her extremely short time frame. Emily has a more realistic and attainable goal and is currently considered overweight with her BMI. Based on her goal and the time frame, she could attain this goal and consider it realistic.

Relevant: As this example illustrates, while this goal is attainable for Mia, is it relevant to her current body? Maybe she doesn't like the shape and wants to be curvier, or she wants to have leaner thighs. Mia needs to relook at what is relevant to her body image that needs to change. Emily could benefit from the same reflection, though her goal appears to be relevant as she is at a higher BMI.

Timely: Mia has a very stringent time frame of 30 lbs. in 4 weeks; this results in a rapid weight loss plan of 7.5 lbs./week. The recommended weight loss is 2–5 lbs./week, based on other factors. Emily has a more sensible plan of losing 5 lbs./week; though still aggressive, it is more relevant to what is realistic. However, it must also be relevant to her own eating habits and exercise plan, as she cannot assume that simply wanting to lose weight (without making any effective changes) can result in reaching her goal.

These two examples look at the SMART goals in a different perspective, but readily demonstrate how we may *think* a goal is SMART but really need more details in order to be SMARTer. If someone came to your class, observed you teaching according to your lesson plan, could they claim you met the goals of the day? Of the lesson plan? Often the objectives are written in such a way as to discern whether the objective was met. Usually written in the context of "as a result of this learning, student will be able to ..." it allows the observer to determine whether the objective was met. But as we stated, sometimes there are more goals than the ones simply written as an objective.

Instruction

What does this word mean to you? Does it refer to your plan, or the method that you teach? Does it refer to the earlier referenced goals and objectives? Note: this word is a noun, not a verb. What is the difference between instruction and learning? Between learning and education? Having a clear understanding of instruction will help you decipher whether you have met the goals for your course. According to various dictionaries, instruction is defined as the action or act of teaching. Learning is what is acquired as a result of instruction. Education is a field of study involving instruction and learning. So back to the question at hand: how do you know if your instruction (art of teaching) is effective? Did students learn something as a result of your instruction? Considering what they learned, was it planned, happenstance, in addition to the goals and objectives, or in lieu of? If you set out to teach them about healthy nutrition and reviewed various diets, but also started discussing basal metabolic rate (BMR) and BMI, perhaps they learned more than what you planned. If your instruction got off course and you discussed disordered eating but did not get to cover the basics of nutrition, you may think your lecture/instruction was effective as learning took place, even though they did not learn what was planned for the day. This is not necessarily a bad thing, as covering eating disorders is part of the overall plan for the course. However, if your students learned how to make a vegetarian lasagna to help them know how to cook healthy (and that is *all* they learned), your instruction was not effective for the purpose of the course or the daily lesson plan. In order to evaluate whether your instruction was effective, you must begin with the end in mind.

In Chapter 7 we will review both formative and summative assessments. These assessments are one way to determine whether you met your goals, and/or the goals set forth by the institution. Ongoing evaluation must take place to see if you are on course, off course and can easily get back on course, or are totally off course and need help. This navigational example is also true for your students in their own learning, as they can just as easily go off on tangents in their learning and steer away from the goals you have in mind. Discussing goals on a weekly or even daily basis is a good way for you and your students to check in and ensure the discussions, activities, and learning that is occurring parallels with the overall goals for the class and the course. While it is acceptable to add to the instructional goals you have been given, you must ensure, at a minimum, you meet the basics.

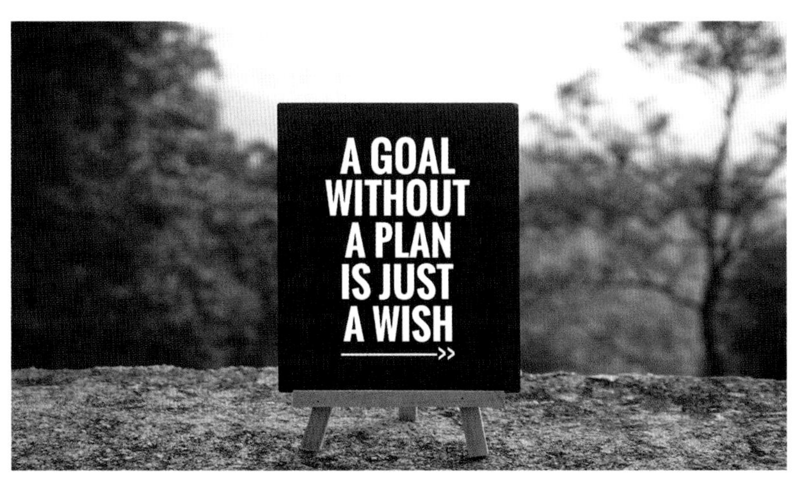

(Coompia77/iStock.)

Another point to consider is whether *your* learning took place? As you were teaching and offering various activities, did you plan enough time, resources, or ensure the students had equal representation? Did you practice enough so that the activity went smoothly? Were there hiccups that could have been prevented? Did you review the material to the point of knowing it without having to look up information or correct yourself? Evaluation of instruction also implies we evaluate the instructor; if you did not present the material in an effective manner, it could impede learning. Self-evaluation is part of determining whether instruction was effective.

How Do You Decide What Is Important?

In order to use the SMART goal planning technique, you must ascertain which items are important to evaluate. For example, is it just as important to have students work together in teams as it is to cover your material? If so, then ice breakers and team building activities are also important. Is it important that students be aware of how to interview and use interpersonal skills in a job search? Then soft skills need to be included in your class in addition to the résumé building. Sometimes the underlying knowledge needs elaboration, and that must be factored in so that students can meet the objectives. If the goals are a bit too high for your students, include some "unofficial" ones to ensure the overall goals are attainable—this is what makes them smart!

There are other ways to ensure you are meeting goals, objectives, and students' goals in learning. One of the most obvious is to ask, informally or formally, such as with student surveys. You can begin to review test scores and determine if indeed most (over 50% of the class) answered correctly. By screening the questions ahead of time, you hopefully were able to catch errors. However, in hindsight, some questions may have been confusing or had two very close answers. Test review is effective both pre- and posttest; however, you also need to scrutinize the results. Students will often want you to throw out a test question, which is usually frowned upon. However, you may inform them that you will review the question to ensure they are learning the material. If after reviewing the test you determine that they really did not understand a particular topic or main point (as evidenced by the fact that no one got that question correct, or less than half of the class did), this becomes a new teaching opportunity. Learning did not take place—for whatever reason, and thus the instruction was not effective.

Every faculty member has situations in which they felt they have covered a topic, only to find a student or even the whole class fared poorly on a test. As always, take this objective information constructively and see where you can augment their learning. Review your lectures and the test to ensure the students do understand and can demonstrate their understanding via the test (or whatever means you have). Perhaps the test did not portray their understanding or was confusing. Maybe the students can explain things better in other ways versus multiple choice responses; could the test be given as a short answer or essay? If it is a skill, did the student simply get the step out of order, but understands how to perform the skill and can return to demonstrate the skill? These are all important pieces when determining whether the instruction was effective and whether all the learning took place. Most of the information you teach will have numerous applications and can be evaluated in a multitude of ways.

Learning Theories

In considering your own learning, and whether you were able to effectively convey the material to the students, did the theorist you choose work? If you are more of a behaviorist and were attempting to use cognitive principles to teach and motivate students, you may have felt out of place or may indeed have struggled with teaching. If Maslow seems far-fetched and the whole idea of learning via different styles seems preposterous, you may have more challenges meeting the needs of the students. While you know that you covered the material and presented it in a few different ways, you may have missed the mark totally. If students don't make the connection it is difficult (if not impossible) to claim that learning has taken place or that your lecture (no matter how wonderful you feel it was) was effective. If everyone failed the test or failed to answer your questions, something is missing. You cannot put it all on the entire class for not studying if you did not facilitate their learning. As mentioned, it does not mean that you have to review every point or each fact, but you must direct their learning—even if it is self-learning.

Consider a class in which there are many terms to learn, perhaps a psychology course that reviews mental illness. Though you do not have time to review the entire *Diagnostic and Statistical Manual of Mental Disorders*, Fifth Edition (DSM-5), you can alert students to focus on five major categories of mental illness and know the primary disorders involved in them. Perhaps you prepare a handout or have students create an outline so they can fill in the blanks. Or you offer one or two of the five categories to jump start them but allow students to complete the rest of the list and complete the disorders associated within these categories. While you are not responsible for providing the entire lecture, you have taken accountability to ensure students are learning the five main categories (which is one of your course objectives). You may also follow up after giving this assignment to ensure they really did their homework. Again, while you did not spend the class time lecturing, you did circle back to make sure the students learned the material and thus are ready for the next level of understanding (and prepared for the test). In this example, your technique and instruction can both be effective, as the self-learning accompanied by the teacher's guidance results in meeting two objectives. Students know the material and gain a sense of self-efficacy, which fosters motivation. Without realizing it, even if you don't subcribe to self-determination theory (SDT), you have supported it.

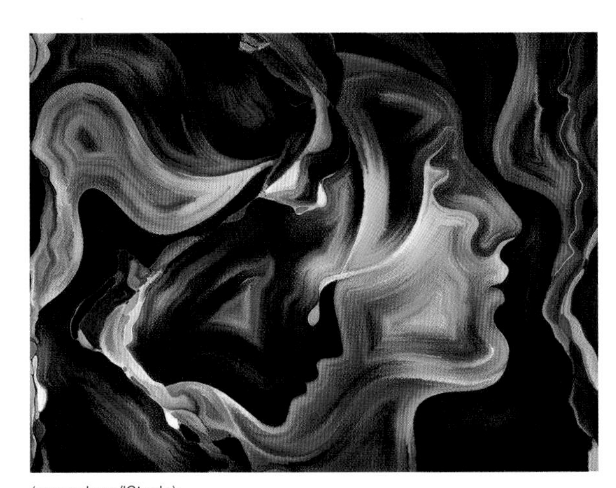

(agsandrew/iStock.)

Bloom's Taxonomy

Recall that Bloom's taxonomy offered various levels for students to learn. As you review each level, you also want to review whether the instruction was effective at each level. Consider back to that class on anatomy. You may need to rethink each level to see where the learning ball got dropped or where students failed to make that connection.

REMEMBERING/KNOWLEDGE

This is the basic level, whereby students learn new terms, new pieces on which to build. You asked students to list or name the major systems of the body, describe each system's function, and list the organs involved. If students became confused, write down the wrong parts, or spell the organs/system incorrectly, they do not have a solid foundation on which to build. If the foundation is off, everything they learn and add to this foundation is moot, as there is not a correct layer on which to add new information. Just like building a house, or a shed, if the subfloor isn't level, your house will be wonky. Go back and reassure yourself they at least could remember basic terms and can recall the appropriate parts. If not, stay on this level until students demonstrate a full understanding of the terms and parts involved. Include other requirements, such as spelling, capitalization, and any other reference points required. Make sure this level is complete by asking students in a variety of ways to answer the question—not necessarily by memorizing the information.

UNDERSTAND

If you assess that indeed they have learned the basics of anatomy, try to recheck with some form of discussion—describe the organ and its function; how it works within the system; how it works with other systems. Review whether they can talk a good talk, or if they can answer some questions and provide more information when you give them a possible scenario. Again, by using the techniques of comparing and contrasting, you should be able to determine if the students are able to demonstrate their understanding. If they stumble, seem confused, or refer to parts that do not make sense or are incorrect, take the time to review this again. You may even take one step back and recall the basic functions and purpose of the organ to remind students how it works and how it works within the body. Pause and reflect on where the students' confusion is stemming from. Getting confused with pulmonary arteries and veins is common as it doesn't follow the "normal" pattern of an artery being oxygen rich and a vein being oxygen deprived. This is what we call a teaching moment—in a very short time you can turn the students' misunderstanding around with a simple clarification, realizing why they got confused in the first place.

APPLY

Reviewing this level requires that the student truly has a grasp of the organs, their function, how they work within the system, and what happens when. They must be able to extrapolate this information into scenarios with basic information—if a student is struggling with any of the prior levels, they will most certainly struggle with applying it to the wider sense of, say, diabetic care. Review the material in smaller chunks to allow them to apply little segments to their learning and determine if they can apply this information in small doses. Your evaluation of learning may need to be at a slower pace to make sure the student isn't jumping from one concept to another. While they may be able to apply the concept of a finger stick to an otherwise healthy diabetic patient, they still get lost when the patient has pancreatic cancer. This is a student who cannot apply these concepts to the overall disease process and needs to review their understanding (previous level).

ANALYZE

If a student truly can recall, understand, and apply these concepts, they should be ready to analyze harder cases. As you review their ability to debate issues and dissect judgment or cases, are they truly getting the gist of the argument? Do they have good rationales to support their opinion or their viewpoint? Can they stand on their own when it comes to defending their ideas? If not, this is a clue that not enough learning has taken place to satisfy this level. Resolve anything that might be confusing the student, such as other viewpoints and personal opinions; in order to be effective, you must allow the student to be seen through a single lens, not one that is joined and blended with other classmates. Instruction cannot be effective if the water is muddy and getting muddier by other students contributing yet more mud. Allow some time to separate those students who clearly do understand and can analyze from those who are still struggling. A lot may also depend on their learning styles, as analytical skills often come easier to the logical learner.

EVALUATE

If indeed the student(s) can analyze, their ability to evaluate should come with some ease. If they know what doesn't belong, for example, they can better ascertain why it *doesn't* and what *does* belong. Being able to differentiate and separate can help students evaluate. However, it is important to remember that evaluation does not necessarily mean judge. Judging, as in discernment, is what we are seeking; judgment, as in rending one's biased opinion, is not. When students judge based on their critical thinking skills, they are looking for what make sense and how it all fits together. This also allows them to broaden their perspective and learning base so they can take on more viewpoints and perpetuate learning. This process can be considered very effective, as we want to instill this lifelong learning concept to students and faculty. If students (or faculty) get to an end point and feel that the thinking process has stopped, ended, or is final, their mind is closed and learning may not continue. This is not effective, as our goal is to always look for new ideas and more information. Education is a journey, not a destination; along the way we want to feed our very hungry minds to seek and discover more. Being able to evaluate allows the learner to sit back, ponder, come up with new information, and determine how it fits in with prior information. Evaluation of new information requires that the learner assimilate this information into what they knew previously. Metacognition takes place and new information is now the baseline for knowledge. However, the faculty's evaluation of this process is still keen. If a student assimilates new information and takes it in to form a new frame of reference, but their perception or evaluation is off, we are continuing with a wonky structure. While the foundation may be stable, the walls and roof aren't. This can happen when a student enters a discussion or debate about a controversial topic, perhaps one that they aren't as familiar with. Despite their literature review and surveys, they may fall short of understanding the bigger picture. Consider a political discussion on prior presidents. Perhaps a discussion is reviewing the popularity of President Barack Obama and President Donald Trump. While there are many differences, there are a few similarities in their style. However, in looking at popularity, there are distinctions in their followers. The naïve students may think that younger voters find President Obama to be a better president and assume they don't like Trump, while thinking that most white males are bigots and love President Trump. Their evaluation of the popularity of these two presidents (regardless of the polls) has failed to consider that millennials only knew one president before Trump (Obama) and thus had only one reference point to compare Trump to (Obama). Though they have read about other presidents, they have had no other personal experience with any other president. On the flip side, perhaps many men like Trump, because they can also relate to his business model, or his tactics. You should not defend either president as to how they connect with their constituents, but rather try to discern the students' ability to evaluate popularity. If your personal viewpoint on either president wedges into the discussion, the students continue to allow biases to impede their ability to evaluate. Instruction is not effective if they use a narrow perspective in which to evaluate.

CREATE

At this level, the student should be able to create a new project or design without prompting, based on all perspectives and angles, without bias. They should be, much like you, open to new ideas and moving forward in their learning. It is often a great sigh of relief for the faculty member when a student can create their own lesson plan or study guide (with answers) correctly. This reinforces that learning took place, the students have achieved each level of the taxonomy, and they truly do know the material. This is best seen when students can offer peer mentoring and can guide other students in their learning. If a student can teach another student with accurate information, you know they have learned; after all, isn't that what you are doing? Evaluation of instruction needs to come at every aspect of learning, as each level can have setbacks, offer opportunities for misinformation, and can have some students able to meet objectives while others are riding along on the coat tails of their peers. Best practices stem from doing the best at each level, and ensuring each student, collectively and individually, is grasping the material at their own pace, with full comprehension. When you realize that at any level there can be misguided learning and mixed messages, you can better realize that using best practices is not simply a one-size-fits-all approach to instruction.

Course Planning

When it comes to evaluating your own teaching, sometimes you must go back to the basics yourself. If your students are not grasping the material or are getting confused, stumped, coming up with wrong answers or conclusions, you may need to reevaluate your own lesson plan. As you reflect on how you planned the lesson, did you consider the needs of your students? Did you allow enough time for the students to ask questions, process the information, or get to each level in Bloom's taxonomy? What about your teaching style—was it effective? Let's take a brief look at some of the pitfalls and ways your teaching style may not have been effective.

- **Lecture:** the least effective overall as students can easily lose interest. How long was your lecture? Was it more of a monologue, without any engagement, or just you talking for long periods of time? Consider doing smaller lectures (less than 30 minutes). Try to review a topic or main point, include various activities (some can be 1–5 minutes) and regroup for additional lectures. Also remember that in order to engage students, they must do something active—lecturing is completely passive, even if they are taking notes. Rethink how you can get your students actively involved and doing something so they can stay focused and maintain some level of interest.
- **PowerPoint (PPT):** like lectures, this is often a very passive way of instruction and one of the less effective ways to get students involved. While you may need to include PPT slides, you must consider how to use them while engaging the student. If you show a few slides and leave out pieces of information, ask the student to fill in the blanks and complete the thought process in their note taking. Active participation does not mean asking the students to read PPT slides—this is just as ineffective as you reading the slides. It requires little interaction and accomplishes less learning. Students may stumble over words and read very slowly; other students are not engaged and can easily be bored. Without some creativity, PPTs and lectures are not considered best practices in teaching due to their lack of student engagement and lack of active learning.
- **Hands on:** depending on your topic, your class preparation should include something that students must use their hands (or body) to do. If you are to get them active, consider getting them physically active as well as mentally active. Did you get them outside, walking or searching—seeking and discovering? Did you include something for them to build, play with, or practice a skill on? Effectiveness in this teaching style will mean having each student work at their own pace and at their level to get to a common point. Perhaps you did a trust walk and everyone had the opportunity to be the leader and the blindfolded person. Maybe your class was on teambuilding in the workforce and you gave them supplies to build a tower or had them play tug-of-war. Even if you did these hands-on activities, were they effective? In retrospect, did the activity go as planned or did it go awry? Did students go off course and do their own thing, or did they end up with different conclusions? While learning took place maybe they did not learn what your objective was. Review this tactic and see what could be done differently; ask students how the exercise could have been changed to accomplish the goal.
- **Videos:** although videos can be great as a short review of a concept or skill, be sure that you don't lose your audience when showing a video. Much like lectures and PPT, it is a passive form of learning. During the video have students listen for answers to a pre-set list of questions (short). Review their answers after the video to make sure they paid attention,

understood, and could reiterate the main concepts. While videos don't rank high with student's engagement, they (when kept brief and including some activity) can be effective. A postanalysis is needed to determine if indeed the video helped or hindered students' understanding of the skills or concept.

- **Guest speakers:** no matter how excited you are to have someone come and speak on your topic, their effectiveness parallels the same principles as lectures and PPTs, videos, and activities as if you were the speaker. Students can enjoy outside speakers, but the same rules of engagement apply. Guest speakers can also introduce material contrary to your lectures and can easily go off on tangents. You may want to interject politely if you see this train wreck coming, or discreetly share after the guest speaker is done that while this information was important and relevant, it is a bit different from what you have shared with students. Note that the guest lecturer was not wrong, but came from a different perspective. You never want to discount the value of outside speakers, as it reflects on you, as the primary person responsible for course planning.
- **Small groups:** while this involves students a great deal, it can also be ineffective if the mix of students doesn't mesh, or if they all agree and thus have no different perspectives. It also is ineffective if they spend their time socializing or if one or two (or the whole group) is quiet. You need to get into each group and ensure they are on topic, dialoguing and staying focused on the activity at hand.
- **Games and puzzles:** nothing deflates the enthusiasm of a creative teacher more than planning an engaging game or activity, only to have the students roll their eyes, go off on other tangents, and refuse to cooperate. Although teaching doesn't come with a crystal ball, you should have tested the waters and tried out a few smaller activities to determine whether an entire class day should be devoted to this game. Smaller games or puzzles can give you a clue as to the interest level, and what you may need to tweak before attempting the activity again. Asking students after a brief game of *Kahoot!* if they liked it (regardless of their involvement) can guide you next time. Maybe it was fun for today, but they'd rather not do it every day. Perhaps they got confused and just followed along, pretending to understand as they played. Maybe you need to go slower to allow those who aren't as savvy with tech games to learn how to play first, before moving on to the subject material. Don't be confused by the smiles on their faces; ask students to determine whether the game was fun and whether they learned. It is possible that the game was fun, but they learned nothing as a result of it.
- **Critical thinking:** while you spent 20 hours on your critical thinking activities you may have missed the point. Relook at what the point was (which can easily get lost while planning these activities). Just as with any other class activity, there must be a goal or objective in mind—did you reach this goal/objective? *Enjoyment* of these activities is the icing on the cake; you need to first ensure whether your cake is well baked. Did the students get the point of the activity? Did they do it on their own (a critical component of thinking)? In Bloom's taxonomy, this activity gets to at least the level of analyzing, so students should be able to begin evaluating whether learning took place as a result of this activity.
- **Case studies:** as with critical thinking exercises, this activity requires analytical skills and the ability to pull abstract facts together to form a deeper understanding and a higher level of thinking. If students cannot pull these abstract pieces together, several things may be missing: the details are too abstract to pull together (teacher need to rethink facts); the student is unable to analyze (need to bring exercise down to applying); and/or the student cannot predict outcomes (teacher needs to rethink thought process or obstacles to learning). Perhaps everyone in the class was able to get through the deductive reasoning on the crying infant example in Chapter 5 except George. In George's culture, men are not involved in the care of children; George does not care if the infant is crying and has no interest in consoling

him. If this were a case study for a psychology course, a class on human or childhood development, George would not participate fully as his reference stems from a very different referenced point. Many cultures have absolute views on parenting, death, the dying process, and the roles of men and women; there is no discussion or opposing viewpoint considered. The cultural stand is finite. Case studies are ineffective if you expect George to support an opposing view, or ask him to debate the opposite side from his beliefs.

- **Debates:** just like case studies, a debate can totally derail a class whereby students are unable to see the other side or support viewpoints outside of their own. Even during a debate, while students are defending their "side," they should be open to other viewpoints. This must be planned in order for the debate to be an effective part of the class discussion. If you have students from various cultures where there is no leeway, you may not want to do a traditional debate, but rather a focused debate. Focused debates allow students to briefly share their side without the expectation that they have an open mind (some might say that political debates are focused debates). Again, prior planning ensures that you have contingencies in place in case the debate becomes heated or the audience (other students) feel offended. It is the audience's responsibility to have the open mind, not the opposing debaters.
- **Independent study:** as much as you want your students to be able to do independent study, some have never learned that way and are lost if you walk away. Be patient with students who seem to cling to traditional instruction; don't nudge them too fast to learn a large amount of material on their own. Start with some simple activities or homework, perhaps even more than the rest of the class, to increase their self-efficacy (to reinforce they *can* learn on their own, without you); let them know you are available if they have questions they absolutely cannot find the answer to. Be sure to have very clear boundaries; otherwise, they might never truly attempt to be independent learners. It is possible to do too much hand holding with students! If you ask students to perform tasks or activities independently too soon in their learning, it can have the reverse effect; students can feel like a failure and stop trying. They may also feel overwhelmed or that you do not care. Reassure them that you are trying to help them learn more on their own, as an adult, and while they may feel lost, you can help them regroup. Reestablish the trust as much as possible but do not let their feelings of inadequacy dominate their ability to learn independently. Your faith in the process of independent learning, coupled with the pace best for your students, will give them the confidence to continue in their learning and reach their goals. For independent learning to be effective, however, it must be at the best rhythm for students independent of one another. This is not the same as group learning.
- **Field trips:** while most students enjoy any opportunity to get out of class, your field trip should have dovetailed into the lecture or activity you reviewed. Whatever hands-on activity the field trip offered, or additional information they were exposed to, it must be in alignment with what you are attempting to teach the students to learn. Also evaluate the logistics: was it too crowded? Was there ample parking and was it free? Did you spend more time getting to the site than you did at the site? Was there an area for picnicking or the ability to buy refreshments? Was it expensive? These logistics can take even a very appropriate field trip to a place where students feel the entire day was a disaster. Consider Disneyland or another large theme park. While many people look forward to going on the rides, seeing the characters, or watching the shows, no one enjoys the lines, the expensive costs of food and beverages, or the large crowds. The fun of being at the theme park can certainly override the long lines and wait time, but that is only when the participant finds value in the trip. For a young teenager who has waited her whole life to go to Disneyland and meet the character Elsa, the fact that she had to wait for 40 minutes is of no consequence. Her older brother, however,

an Anaheim resident, has been to Disneyland so many times that he cringes in the parking lot. Though he agreed to take his sister and is pleased she enjoys the park, he does not find much value in seeing Elsa or riding the *Star Wars* rides any more. Although your field trip may not equate to Disneyland, did it interest all of your students? Did you scrutinize the logistics to decrease wait times, or ensure there were funds for snacks and beverages? Did you provide value to the field trip, such as asking for a commemorative pen or other suitable token to give students? Students love freebies, and even though they are adults, they appreciate some sort of acknowledgment for their learning. Again, asking students what "treats" or incentives they value is important before you find all their treats in the trash.

Classroom Management

Part of evaluating best practices is in reviewing your own self in the classroom. If your activities were in alignment with your lecture or the information you presented, how was the class? Did you find everyone sitting on the edge of their seats, fully engaged? Or did students get up and walk out on the activity, go to the restroom, or go get a snack? Did you have a lot of interruptions? Were the interruptions because students wanted to get you off topic, or did they ask so many questions because their understanding was muddled?

Student Engagement

Each of these points has referenced the importance of student engagement. However, engagement does not mean that the activity was effective. In fact, the most effective way to determine best practices in student engagement is the student. At the risk of sounding redundant, if students are engaged but not learning, then learning is not occurring. Engaged students, just as in the field trip, may find the activity fun and may participate, but it does not imply they are learning or that they are reaching their goals. Just as correlation does not mean causation, faculty cannot expect that just because students are happy, they understand the activity, the lesson, or the material.

Rethinking Your Practices

In each of the phases of your course planning, classroom management, student engagement activities, and overall critical thinking activities, you must evaluate what worked and what didn't. This often requires that you continuously evaluate your teaching, as best practices occur on a daily, even hourly basis. Identifying best practices is an ongoing pursuit—you will never reach an end point to knowing what works. You can, however, add to your toolbox the variations of each phase in your teaching to provide caveats to activities, and plan for the what if's.

When you consider best practices, and effective instruction, do you personalize this and use it to gauge how well you *performed* in your teaching? Best practices don't necessarily relate to how well we *perform*, but rather *how* well our performance worked. Much like the assessments we will review in Chapter 7, we want to make sure that all your course planning and activities actually reach the student and assist in their learning. If students don't learn, then we need to use different practices. The objective of our teaching is to assist the student in learning, not simply give them great information.

Academic Freedom

While your goals and objectives, as well as some lesson plans, may be given to you by your institution there are other things that you can have input on. These areas, however, are unique to each institution and must be clarified. Some faculty feel that they have freedom to teach whatever they want, however they want, whenever they want. This is not necessarily true, although you may have leniency based on your institution's guidelines. As mentioned in Chapter 2, you do have to adhere to guidelines set forth by your institution, as they have been reviewed and approved by regulatory agencies. While you cannot change goals and objectives, you may be able to change deadlines or the calendar of when activities are done, such as tests. You may not control the end point, but you may have the freedom to change how you get to the end point. If you have your finger on the pulse of your students' learning, you may be better equipped to negotiate freedom in defense of your students.

Keep in mind however, that just as you expect your students to learn the goals and objectives within a certain time frame, your institution expects you to teach to the goals and objectives within that same time frame. While the institution may support your creativity, they may not support changing the framework of the course. This is especially true if more than one faculty member teaches the same course, as it becomes difficult to evaluate overall best practices of multiple classes or instructors as there is no consistency or a common denominator between courses. Much like comparing apples to oranges, if the only thing in common is that they are a fruit, then there is no rationale to support that your way of teaching is more effective than another.

Get Out of Your Own Way

As mentioned in Chapter 3, faculty can exude many personalities or behaviors. Many times, these behaviors stem from an underlying feeling that we must be better prepared, more of a teacher, and smarter than our students. Faculty may feel overwhelmed or underprepared—or even have a notion that they are *supposed* to feel this way. The sense of martyrdom and sacrifice seems to be just part of the job but can truly get in the way of one's success. Wherever these feelings of inadequacy originate, it is important to recognize them for what they are and get out of the way of these negative forces.

You may also find that the course or class ended up meeting the goals regardless of your input. For example, you may have doubted whether the thought exercise in Chapter 4 to compare/contrast Darth Vadar and Mufasa would appeal to all your students, given their different interests and ages. You may have failed to recognize how the activity could help students look outside the box and use critical-thinking skills to be objective. However, your students were able to find similarities as well as differences in the two leaders. They came up with an impressive list of leadership characteristics, teaching them what makes a great leader. The students were able to create the list even though you may have doubted they could put aside any personal differences and come together as a group to compare/contrast fictional characters. Because we are human, we need to know when we are getting in the way of our student's learning and step aside. While it may seem counterproductive, getting out of your own way can be extremely effective and is a very good practice.

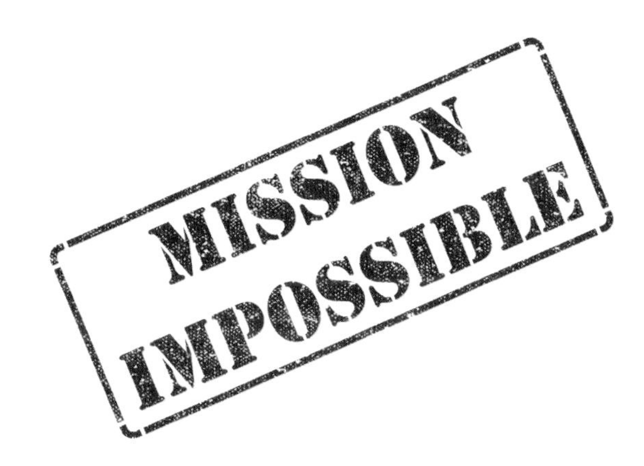

(Tashatuvango/iStock.)

Help Yourself

While you are often your own worst enemy, you can also be your own best friend. Make notes for yourself or guide yourself using PPT slides to prompt you but not to teach for you. Make certain you take time for self-care; there is only one of you and only 24 hours in a day. When you wish there were more than 24 hours in a day, realize you would fill that time with even more things on your to-do list. Slow down and make sure you understand each aspect, especially if it is your first time reviewing a concept or practice. If you have never put together a syllabus, look at one that is well organized and compare it to another faculty members—if you were the student, which pieces would you find important? What else would you want to know?

No one has all of the answers, but chances are there are other faculty (they may even be in another department) that seem to have it all put together. Perhaps they score highly on satisfaction surveys or seem to be calm even if they are teaching multiple classes. Sit down and learn what *their* best practices are. Always add others' practices to your toolbox as an option but remember that their students are not your students. Be sure to do a trial run on your students *before* you accept this activity as a tried-and-true, fail-safe endeavor.

Tricks of the Trade

The adage "fake it till you make it" can often be seen in teaching. You want you assure your students you know what you are doing, even if you feel you don't. Two other adages are "don't let them see you sweat" and "don't sweat the small stuff." While you may be nervous your first day (or first year), know that you will improve if you have an open mind, and you will overcome the hurdles. Just as your students will learn, you will also learn about how to teach, what works, what you are good at, and what doesn't work for you or your students. Be patient—you weren't hired because you know all the answers. You were hired to teach; as teachers, we are also learners.

Every seasoned teacher has a toolbox full of tricks; things they can use at any given time to help defuse a situation. Whether it is an unruly class, a class that lacks motivation, or a class that feels intimidated by the material, there are things they can do to regroup and get back on track. They may even be known as the one who loves to show old movies or hits from the 1980s. What they are attempting to do is have a common place for students to meet without fear or judgment. Maybe they bring in arts and crafts, read a children's short story, or play an unrelated game. Whatever it is, students find themselves more open to learning as a result of this activity. This is a bit different than student engagement, as it simply gives them a time to be human and for you to push the reset button. Brief, fun or silly, and easily introjected, these activities will become part of your repertoire as you become more comfortable (and less critical) of your teaching style.

Checks and Balances

While Chapter 7 will focus on assessments, remember the easiest form of checks and balances is to simply ask your students how they are doing. Are they learning? Is the pace good? Do they still have questions? How do they feel the class is going so far? While you are not necessarily opening yourself up to the minor criticisms that may come from immature or inexperienced students, you are asking for students to offer constructive feedback. Again, take this with a grain of salt. Some of it may seem brutal (do you know anything about our generation?), some may make sense (I'd prefer to take the test closer to the subject, instead of a month later), and some may seem out of your control (why do we really have to stay here for 8 hours?). See if others feel the same way, if it is something worth investigating, or if you indeed have any control over the situation. Always recognize a student's input, address or acknowledge it, and what the resolution is. You may not know much about the current generation (until you read Chapter 8) but can ask that students share with you some information that could help. And while you may be able to schedule the test closer to the time the material was covered, you may not. Explain what you can do and why you may not be able to reschedule that test ("actually there is more to the subject that we need to review that will be on the test; however, I understand your concern and will ensure we do a thorough review before the test to cover older material"). You can relate to their concern ("yes, 8 hours seems like a long day") but don't try to connect too personally ("If I have to be here you have to be here—all 8 hours. I don't like it any more than you do!"). Never fault the administration, your manager, or the institution, as you will create a false ally with students. Moreover, it is never your job to be their buddy; you are the teacher.

Don't Take It Personally

Even though we know students don't (usually) mean to hurt our ego, teachers often feel wounded when students do not like their teaching techniques. They may show it outwardly, may provide negative feedback on a survey, or may request another teacher. They may enjoy your substitute more than they enjoy your class. Regardless of what they say, don't assume you are doing something wrong. What you *are* doing, however, may not be effective. While this is not a time for true confessions, you can ask why they enjoyed the substitute teacher. What was it about that class that was fun? You may discover that the substitute let them out 30 minutes early or provided snacks for them midday. You should thank students for any honest feedback and see if it is in alignment with how you want to teach. Though you would not discount the teacher who allowed them to leave early, you can remind students that you want to ensure you cover the material in the given time so they can be successful on the test. When students realize you have their best interest at heart, they are less likely to be critical of your tactics.

Compare and Contrast

Students are notorious for pooling together and playing one faculty member against another. Perhaps it is human nature, or maybe they feel that they are missing out. Regardless, keep in mind that this occurs and don't fall for it. "But Mr. Right Teacher always lets us do ..."; "Why don't you do this like Ms. Great Teacher?" In this instance, students hone their comparing and contrasting skills with ease and perfection. While your inner child wants to claim "I'm the teacher, that's why," realize that this will ensure a battle of wills and accomplish nothing. Make notations of Mr. Right Teacher and Ms. Great Teacher, letting students know that you will follow up on these suggestions and ask these teachers more about their teaching styles. Students may back off if they consider the other teachers were using ineffective instruction and poor practices (such as releasing students early) to achieve better survey results or to decrease their workload. Never let students know or believe there is any retaliation or reprimand for their sharing; simply thank them for their information.

No doubt, even if your students have not measured you up against other faculty, you probably have done it to yourself. How do you measure up? What is different between you and other faculty? Do you see yourself in their light? Do you feel you are better, or not as good? How many years have they been teaching? Hopefully by the time you have a few classes you have taught and evaluated, you can determine your own best practices, gleaned from others and added their best practices to your toolbox, and no longer scrutinize yourself harshly. We are always improving, practicing, but never will reach perfection. Remove it from your expectations.

Regulatory Agencies and Benchmarks

In addition to your own standards, you will probably have to reach other goals set by agencies such as a board, accreditor, or review committee. You may be evaluated on meeting overall goals and objectives, student surveys, and how your results compare to other teachers nationally. While this can be a humbling experience, it is helpful to see your contribution to education on a grander scale. You may not be aware that your school achieves a higher pass rate on state exams, or that students from your institution are 80% more likely to get a job in their field within 60 days after graduation. Check with other departments, such as Career Services or Student Services, to determine what your benchmarks are. This information, though possibly shared during an admission process, also encourages your students to pursue their own educational goals. It is exciting for them to know that their hard work will pay off if the graduates before them have reached these benchmarks and found jobs within their industries. It also fuels their energy as they realize that they are in this endeavor with others who are looking after them in addition to their teacher. They may not have such backing at home and can feel comforted by this support.

Summary

Best practices will require that you do your own critical thinking and look around you, outside of yourself, and consider your students to determine what part of your instruction is effective. Oral feedback, surveys, test scores, and various other assessments will give you a hint. In Chapter 7, we will use these clues to form an overall systematic method to evaluate our success further through assessments.

Journal—Self-reflection

In the following reflection exercises, consider what you have learned thus far and what you plan on doing as a result of this learning. Whether you have taught courses before, are teaching in a new setting, or have never taught before, you can use this information to shape your class into a better experience—for you and your students.

1 Define the terms according to your own interpretation.

a. Best:

____
____
____
____

b. Practices:

____
____
____
____

c. Effective:

____
____
____
____

d. Instruction:

____
____
____
____

2 What are two goals you have for yourself to improve your teaching, or ensure you are effective with your instruction? List them separately as SMART goals.

a. Goal #1:

S______________________________
M______________________________
A______________________________
R______________________________
T______________________________

b. Goal #2:

S______________________________
M______________________________
A______________________________
R______________________________
T______________________________

c. List three things that can get in your way of achieving these goals.

3 What's most important in your instruction? What are your priorities when teaching? Name at least four things that will be important for you to carry out as you are planning and executing your class.

4 Time to play devil's advocate. If you were watching yourself teach according to Bloom's taxonomy, or in anticipation of how you have planned to teach each level, what is missing? What do you anticipate may not work? Consider each level—what has the teacher planned? What can go wrong? How might this activity not reach the students? Be critical, but compassionate. Don't get down on yourself, rather be constructive about how you can be better. Best practices come from trial and error. You may make adjustments before you ever get to teach that class! Another way of thinking about it is to consider what could go wrong with each level.

a. Remember:

b. Understand:

c. Apply:

d. Analyze:

e. Evaluate:

f. Create:

5 Do the same exercise for classroom management; consider what you haven't planned for yet, or how your planning may not be fail safe.

a. What other possibilities could creep up and get your class off course?

b. How will you overcome this? What can you do now to anticipate this and be better prepared?

6 Getting out of your own way seems like a hard thing to do, but imperative if you are going to be successful.

a. What biases, judgments, or opinions do you have that may conflict with your class or the subject you plan on teaching?

b. What expectations do you have of your students that may be biased, such as expecting them to listen, follow along, do what they are instructed to do? List at least four.

7 Taking care of yourself has already been covered, but as we get deeper into best practices, there may be more that you must do in order to get out of your own way and care for yourself. Teachers must have a tough skin but a tender heart. How will you address this within yourself? What are five specific examples you will use to make sure you are not taking things personally and remain objective, reflective, and continuously improve?

8 Teachers flock together to support one another. Who do you have as a mentor, friend, or role model that you can go to for support, encouragement, or an unbiased viewpoint of your instruction?

9. As we have covered six chapters, perhaps you have learned a few things that you did not know prior to starting this process. Write a few things down that have helped you; these may be areas where you did not realize you needed to improve but have a better chance knowing that you are armed with more information.

10. Lastly, write a few words of encouragement for yourself. When the tough days come, reflect on these words from your heart to keep *you* motivated.

Chapter 7

Assessments

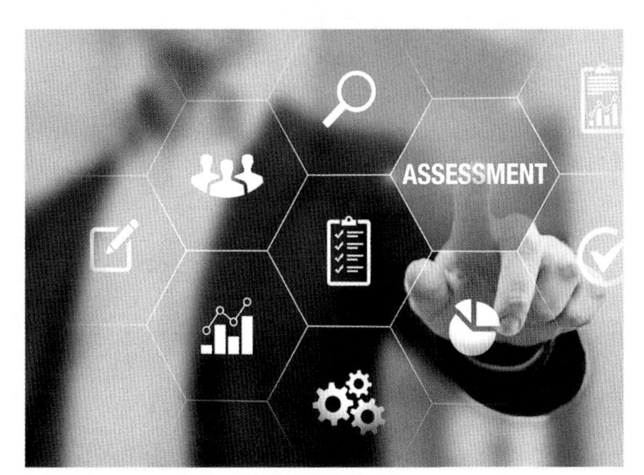

(NicoElNino/iStock.)

Following up on best practices, we now cover formal assessments, or evaluations. "Evaluate" is the fifth step in Bloom's taxonomy and requires that faculty, as the guides of instruction, have a thorough understanding of the overall process of learning. This implies that faculty are clear on what the concept/material is (curriculum design), the execution (instruction), and what the outcomes should be (goals and objectives). It takes into consideration that evaluation is an ongoing process, and that we must look at each step along the way to determine whether we are on course. As you have planned your course, are you reaching the points you created along the way? Are your students able to meet these points as well? Can they incorporate each level of Bloom's taxonomy? At the end of your instruction (class or course), how will you know if the students were able to comprehend or learn the material? How can you assess this learning? If you are off track, how will you regroup so that you still have an opportunity to facilitate learning? While course planning is one of the most important aspects in instruction, evaluation is just as important as it offers you, the faculty member, an opportunity to edit your plan as needed. In preparing for assessments, we must know what to evaluate, when to evaluate, how to evaluate, and what to do with the evaluation results. As with previous chapters, we start at the end.

What to Evaluate

Before you get your red pen out ready to correct every mistake, let's consider what we need to evaluate and why. While it may seem obvious, there are many things you may not have to evaluate even if they are not correct. It is often challenging for the eager faculty member to realize not every wrong answer must be accurate. Just as with teachers, we are not requiring students to be perfect. We are expecting that they meet the goals and objectives and may learn a few more things along the way. However, we still allow them to be human, creative, and have their own opinions, feelings, and perspectives (which may seem biased, but are never wrong). We also allow leniency when we allow students to defend their own learning and accept that multiple goals may be reached in certain situations. When we assess, evaluate, or gauge an assignment, we must focus on the assignment, not the student. We are not judging how smart they are, how well they learn, or how appropriate their answers are. We must focus on what we are evaluating and whether the student's *actions* reached the expectation. Of course, there are times when we assess student's behavior (as discussed in Chapter 2 classroom management); for purposes of this chapter, however, we will only focus on performance.

Goals, Objectives, and Outcomes

One of the most obvious ways to ensure you are effective in your teaching is to determine whether the goals, objectives, or outcomes were met. However, there is a slight difference in these terms, despite the fact that they are often (erroneously) used interchangeably. Goals are written in a very general language, toward an overall achievement. Often the goal is long term, such as being a better student or a better teacher. While the goal may not be easily defined (what does "better" look like?), the objectives are measurable. Goals are broad based; objectives are detail oriented; the steps needed to get the student to the goal. Goals can follow the SMART (specific, measurable, attainable, relevant, timely) method and be specific, but objectives are even more specific. Outcomes are even more precise than the objectives. As a result of reaching the objectives, students will be able to know some information or perform a skill. As you can imagine, the semantics can be very confusing. Usually instructional designers and curriculum development gurus have done this fine tuning for you, but let's review terms that can assist you as you gain more knowledge on assessments.

Let's consider a class on heart health. The goal of the class is to introduce students to behaviors and lifestyles that contribute to a healthy heart. This goal is very generic, broad based, and can be used in a variety of courses such as anatomy, physiology, pathophysiology, and nutrition, for an even wider variety of students in health care (medicine, nursing, dental, physical therapy), physical education (PE), social and behavioral therapies, and the study of spirituality (mindfulness, yoga, meditation). The objectives will be geared toward the students in that discipline and may be different. For example, classes for nursing students will be slightly different from that for PE students. While both courses may cover diet, exercise, and stress, the objectives in the nursing course will have outcomes that relate specifically to hypertension, cardiac monitoring, and heart health based on anatomy and physiology, disease process, and medications. The PE students will focus more on exercise and diet, with little introduction to disease process and will never touch on medications. The outcomes also will vary, as nursing students will have skills related to heart health, such as blood pressure (BP), pulse (apical and radial), and electrocardiograms (ECGs); the PE students may know how to take a pulse, but not know the advanced skills that nursing class covered.

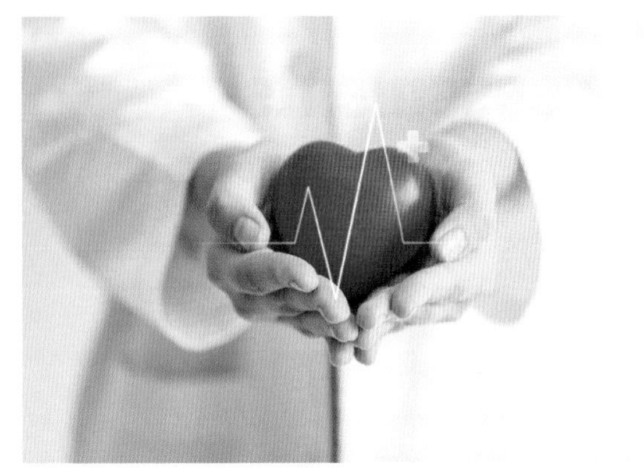

(Peera_Sathawirawong/iStock.)

When assessing goals, objectives, and outcomes, your syllabus should clearly delineate what should be accomplished. This provides your framework for monitoring and will answer many questions when evaluating students' work. Perhaps your class objectives include being able to list five prominent factors that contribute to the risk of heart failure and to identify the role that fats play in the diet. The outcome (as a result of this class) is that you have your students design a low-fat meal for a vegetarian. Consider our example in Chapter 6: if a student knows how to make a low-fat vegetarian lasagna but does not understand how fat increases the risk of heart failure, then the student did not reach the objective, despite the fact they could perform the basic task. If they were able to discern which fast foods support low-fat diets and what store brands are better than others, that's great! But it still does not reach the objective.

How to Evaluate

In the previous example, you would want to note that the student had great ideas and provide positive feedback, but also explain why they received a zero for their assignment. Sometimes students have a difficult time staying focused on the objective and may need guidance, or they may not be incorporating each level of Bloom's taxonomy. Sometimes the objectives may not be understood by the student, despite your many reviews of the assignment. However, while these aspects are noteworthy, you are assessing whether learning has taken place based on the objectives and outcomes as identified in the syllabus.

Knowing *how* to evaluate is a key aspect in assessing a student's learning. Feedback, grades, and scores provide information to the student to direct their learning as the student is wondering whether they are reaching the objectives and the overall goal (though their goal and objectives might be different). Perhaps their goal is to use this class to get to a better paying job, and their objective is to simply pass with a "C" or better. They may focus their studying on only knowing what is on the test and even continuously ask the question whether your material will be on the test. It is not your role to evaluate the student's motivation to pass the course, or to get a better paying job. Your focus is strictly on the work they submit and if it meets the criteria to earn points or accomplish the objective. Though you may give feedback, it must be constructive according to the requirements of the assignment. For instance, you cannot state: "if you put more effort into this homework you could have earned an 80%, which will help you in the next class." You can state "there are three missing aspects to the assignment based on the rubric: you did not relate to how saturated fats contribute to heart risk, how a high-fat diet can increase the risk of heart attacks, nor provide a sample vegetarian meal for a patient at risk. Understanding these principles can help you further when you take advanced nutrition, as you will be expected to master these concepts."

How to Measure Learning

When evaluating an assignment, there is more than one way to assess whether learning has occurred. The most obvious is whether you can grade it or give it a score. If you can give a grade, what is it based on? If someone else had to grade the assignment, would they offer the same score? Is there a place whereby you decide what is worth points or what is not important? This is where rubrics are important. It also falls back on your objective and outcomes, as there may be other ways to ascertain the student learned something, such as check offs for skills, reports or essays (verbal or written), or creation of a project.

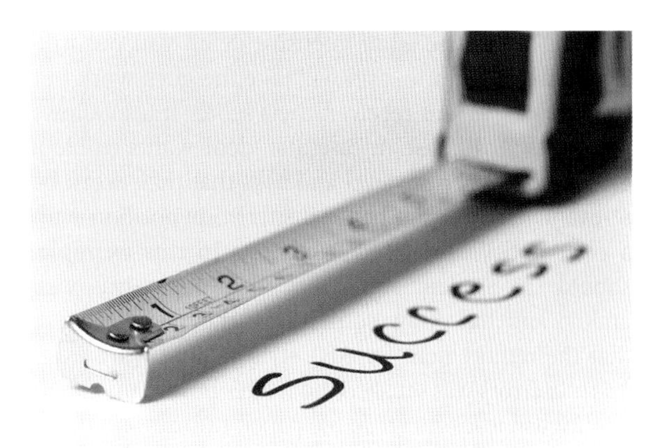

(ImageDB/iStock.)

Rubrics

Rubrics are score cards and can be easily created, copied, and edited based on your criteria. They may come with a preset course complete with objectives, or you may have to create your own. The rubric can be created in Microsoft Word or Excel and resembles a table. Usually there are four or five categories (columns) on a scale of performance, such as exceptional or outstanding, good, satisfactory or acceptable, poor or unacceptable. Each row matches the criteria you are evaluating. For example, one criterion for a four-page writing assignment could be "Written in American Psychological Association (APA) format with proper grammar, sentence structure, and spelling." Each column has points based on how well the student was able to meet this objective:

- Exceptional or outstanding = two or fewer errors
- Good = three or four errors
- Satisfactory or acceptable = five or six errors
- Poor or unacceptable = more than six errors

If a student asks why they received zero points for this category, anyone can refer to the eight various spelling and grammatical errors, as well as the fact that the paper was written in 18-point font single spaced. Clearly this paper was not in APA style and over the "limit" of spelling and grammatical errors, thus the students received zero points.

There are many rubric creator software programs and websites; though often tedious the first few times, it is important to invest the energy as you (and your students) will refer to this as the "holy grail" of points. You will appreciate the labor-intensive detail you put into a well-created rubric, as it will take the guesswork out of why the student received their score. It also allows the basis for defense in case a student wants to file a grievance to the next level and asks that their work be re-evaluated. You can better justify your position with a clear and well-defined rubric. As in this example, should the student argue that their paper was well crafted and full of awesome ideas, they cannot argue that the requirement for APA style writing with fewer than six errors was satisfied, no matter how many different English teachers grade the paper. Rubrics should be handed out along with the syllabus, or at the very least when the assignment is given. The rubric will guide the student on what to focus on and also how to complete the project. Perhaps one of your criteria is to cite three peer-reviewed references; students know they must use the library and not just the Internet to find appropriate literature for their paper. However, another class on current events may not require a literature review and instead ask that students use more contemporary Internet sites and social media to find current topics to support their viewpoint. Though rubrics should not be too specific, they need to be very clear.

Return Demonstration/Check-off

Sometimes a rubric is not necessary as the task itself can determine whether the student met the objective. This is primarily true when there is a specific skill that the student must demonstrate or if they must perform a task. If you are asking students to measure BP using a manual sphygmomanometer (BP cuff) and you have specific placement sites for the cuff and the stethoscope and will obtain the reading yourself to compare for accuracy, no rubric is needed. Perhaps you allow ±5 mm for the reading: if the student places the cuff and stethoscope correctly and obtains a 140/75 and you obtain a 142/76, the student has met the criterion for that skill. Just as with a rubric, however, your expectation of each step must be clear. If you did not include placement of the cuff or stethoscope in your expectations, for example, and simply stated the students must come up with a BP ±5 mm of your reading, students will not focus on correct placement. While you know this can alter the reading and result in an inaccurate BP, your students are simply doing what you asked—taking a measurement.

Test/Quizzes

Based on the material covered, you may be using tests and quizzes as part of your assessments. While it may seem that tests are the easiest form of assessment, they can be quite complicated based on the type of test you are administering. Tests must also make up a percentage of the overall score or grade for the course, as outlined in your syllabus. Perhaps you have eight tests in a 2-month course; that is one test every week. If you are not preparing your students for this rigor, they can easily fall behind, especially if there is also a mid-term and/or a final. Are the weekly test cumulative, or just a comprehensive mid-term and final? Cumulative means that all the preceding chapters or information is included; a comprehensive final includes material from day one. A final that is not comprehensive starts with material covered right after the mid-term. This makes a huge difference for students who are studying, as well as the faculty member as they are preparing a review of the material (you need to know what to include in your review). However, these decisions should have already been made and included in your syllabus based on the curriculum.

Tests come in various formats and with varying question styles. Some material is better assessed with open-ended questions or short essays, such as "What is your perspective on the current climate of homelessness in our region?" You would want your students to cite what is currently being done as well as the plight of homelessness in your area. Students could render their opinion, but it also must be based on some review of current trends and information. Another example is to ask students to create a sample plan for the care of an unwed 13-year-old pregnant teenager. These social concerns cannot easily be fit into a multiple-choice question, as there are varying pieces to the answer. If you felt the need to incorporate a multiple-choice question, you could ask which agency is most likely to assist this teenager and offer four options (of which only one is correct). Be cautious when asking short answer and open-ended questions; if there is a short response (such as "no" or "because it is the law") you will not get the robust response desired. Rubrics of some sort are also needed for these answers and should be clear. If you ask the student to list three resources for that unwed teenager, and they list two, how many points do they get? (Note: they cannot receive more points by citing six resources.)

Other formats of questions can be via true, false, reverse true/false, fill in the blanks, and matching. True/false questions should be very clear, with no exceptions. A question that reads "there are four chambers of the normal heart" is true; the emphasis is on the world *normal*. Are there ever situations whereby there are five chambers in a heart? Yes, in cor triatriatum, a rare disease in infants. However, normal hearts have only four chambers. This question can also be made into a false statement and a reverse true/false. In reverse true/false, the student must first delineate whether the statement is true or false, and if false, make it true. For example: "there are three chambers of the normal heart." The student must first claim this statement is false, and cross out "three" and put "four" to make it true. This test question can also be posed as a fill-in-the-blank question: "there are _____ chambers of the normal heart." If you want to get into the various chambers, you can have a matching or labeling exercise whereby students must match the right and left atria and ventricles to their correct location.

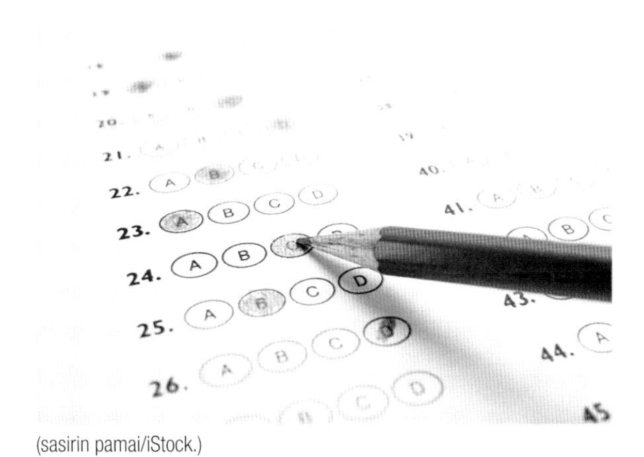

(sasirin pamai/iStock.)

In addition to the style and format of questions is how you will execute the tests. More tests are being conducted online, via the book's publisher, a preparatory program, or via one of the institution's software programs. Some of these programs will do the grading and allow you, as faculty, to edit it. Others require that you do all the work but offer guidance, such as similar answers. Some institutions use paper and pencil tests, Scantrons, or require you to create a document. Whatever setting is used to take the tests must be taken into consideration, especially for the student who suffers from test anxiety.

If it is not differentiated in your syllabus, you will need to decide if you want to add quizzes, pre-posttest, and open book tests. These may be for points (if included in your syllabus thus your expectations) or may be used as a review, indicating there are no points per se. These assessments can be quite instrumental as they are often seen as nonthreatening. Students can use them as a guide for their own learning, to determine what they are knowledgeable about, and where they may still be unclear. Faculty can also use this as the litmus test of understanding and gauge their additional instructions accordingly. These can be take home, open book, or pop quizzes, based on your objective. They should be mandatory (even if they are not worth points) and can be used as a ticket to return to class. Students often need some "requirement" in order to take accountability and complete an assignment worth no points or grade.

Testing Environment

Some institutions use the same premise as national exams (e.g., ACT, SAT, GRE—standardized tests used for college admissions) when it comes to testing environments. Students must have an ID, no cell phone, no notes or anything to create notes, no purse/bags or other materials allowed in the testing room, and no breaks (or only scheduled breaks at certain times). If your students must comply with this environment, make sure you review this ahead of time. These restrictions, though valid and for good reason, can increase anxiety. Being that many students already suffer from test anxiety, the more comfortable they are with the environment the better as it can aid in performance.

Concerns in the testing environment may stem from the opportunity students have to cheat or look at other students' answers, search for answers (especially in a computer-based test), or delay answering. If a student cannot take a test today because they are sick, and asks to postpone it until the next day, they may be waiting to get the answers from another student who took the test today. Assuming you will give the same test to the sick (now miraculously cured) student as the rest of the class, you have compromised the integrity of the test and allowed the recovered student an unfair advantage. Cheating can occur in other forms, such as the old-fashioned passing notes, tapping (who says Morse code is outdated?), and looking at one another's answers. Students can buy tests online through a variety of websites (often for less than $20) and hire others to write their papers. With so much reliability being compromised, what is a teacher to do?

Make sure you are walking around the testing room (if possible), looking casually at where students are looking. While you don't want to hover over them and create undue suspicion, you do want to see if their eyes are wandering, if they appear to be thinking, or if their eyes are darting toward some clues. Have a few additional questions or edit the questions on tests from prior classes, even for the student who was sick. While the material must be the same, the questions (and answers) do not have to be. Students can memorize "correct" answers but will struggle with answering the question if the format is different. If the first test asked how many chambers are in a normal heart, and the makeup test asked to list the chambers of the heart, the students taking the makeup test would stumble if they did not honestly study. Although you don't want to purposely make a test hard or cause confusion, you do want to ascertain whether the student has learned that the normal heart has four chambers and can reveal this knowledge honestly and independently of other students.

Test Analysis

Despite the time and energy, you, or your test prep company, put into creating the test, there may be errors. Always review a test prior to administering it, after administering it, and more than once if possible. During these reviews you will ensure you have (or will) covered the material and that you have the same answers that are on the test. In Chapter 2 it was mentioned that teaching to the test is frowned upon but teaching to the material covered in the test is essential. If the test asked students to label all four chambers of the heart, plus the pulmonary artery/vein, the aorta, all of the valves, and the flow of the heart, then this is much more than what you covered (only the four chambers). Another example is in the question "Which valve is between the left atrium and left ventricle?" The choices are bicuspid, tricuspid, aortic, and pulmonary; the correct answer is bicuspid, otherwise known as the mitral valve. However, you never included the term bicuspid valve in your lectures, only the term mitral. You would catch this on a pretest analysis and quickly remind students (during a test review or when teaching the class) of the two synonymous terms. If it wasn't caught before the exam, you may choose to alert students to this during the test. If, in a worst-case scenario, you didn't catch the term "bicuspid," it may be found in your posttest analysis.

After your test is administered, review the answers and which questions students got wrong. If possible (as with electronic tests), determine what percentage of the students erred on the question. If more than half of the class got a question wrong, was there another answer that appeared to be more correct? While your institution may not allow you to change or edit the test or the results, you can learn from this analysis the next time you cover this material. Perhaps you will go into more detail or pay closer attention to some of the facts to ensure students do not get confused the next time you teach this class. If your institution policy allows you to grant credit if the test question was confusing or the answer options were wrong, be careful how you share this (if you choose to) with students. If students feel that every question is negotiable on the "correct" answer, you will spend more time listening to their arguments of why they should get credit for the wrong answer than you will providing the material for the topic. Many faculty have steered away from discussing correct answers; they instead review what content was missed and where students need to focus. There should be consideration for students who wish to come to you and review their test; if your policy is that students cannot review their exact test (for purposes of integrity) offer similar questions to determine why they do not understand the content. Many students will discover they knew the material; however, they changed their answers, second-guessed themselves, or rushed through their test. Often reviewing effective test-taking skills is needed to help these students be more successful in improving their test scores.

Discussions/Essays/Papers

As mentioned, discussions, essays, and other papers are great ways to determine a student's knowledge on a specific topic. These types of assignments should be reserved for moments when there are details and facts (to ensure for accuracy) and/or can include a personal analysis. Because a rubric is necessary, you must be clear what the objective is in writing this essay/paper or what the discussion/presentation is geared toward. For example, the essay on "What is your perspective on the current climate of homelessness in our region?" must include specific data on your region, what percentage of the population are homeless, and how it may affect your region (jobs, housing, attraction for tourisms/visitors, etc.). If, for example, your region does not have a homeless population, there is no purpose in writing the paper. If the student only offers a personal viewpoint and fails to recognize the impact on the region, then the rubric should illustrate a loss of points. Students must know what to expect so they can begin with the overall picture and not have to piecemeal along the way.

Teacher
Grade Scale
A 90-100%
B 80-89%
C 70-79%
D 60-69%
F 0-59%
CONTENT AR

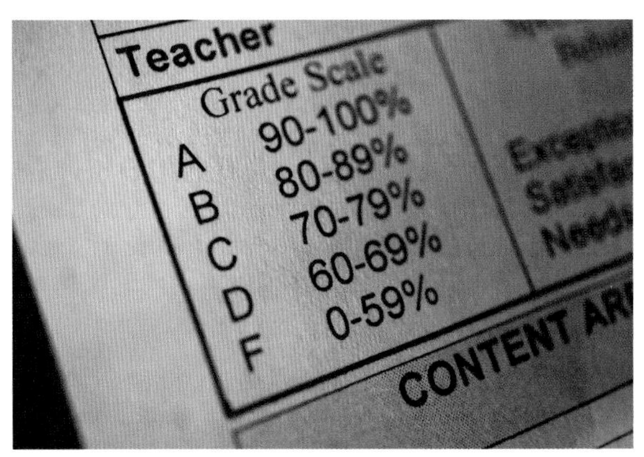

(Kameleon007/iStock.)

Grades

Though we hope that one day students will simply enjoy the class for the sheer pleasure of learning, most are focused on their grade. That also means they will defend their grade, or what they feel their grade should be. Which also means you must defend why you gave the student the grade they received. Simply stating they "earned it" does not suffice. *If* you were not there, can someone else offer a grade? And if so, would it be the *same* grade? This is where your rubrics are crucial, as well as what is in your syllabus. If, for example, you state that students receive a zero for late work, then all late work should earn zero points. *If* you ever deviate from that and allow one student to receive *any* points for late work, you have negated your syllabus. In order to be fair, you must be consistent.

In reviewing grades, there can be no subjective information; it must always be based on objective data. Based on the syllabus and rubric, assignment, or checklist, students receive points. If they do not do what is expected, they receive no points. If it is this cut and dried, it makes is more definitive for students and ensures there is equality in grading, which is what we want. There should never be a situation whereby some students receive points based on personal interpretation or your perception, or that you like "these" students and know they have a better intention. All students are treated equally, and thus, fairly. If you make an exception for one student, you must make it for all. If a student is confused on the syllabus because of the holiday and thought Thursday was the test day, instead of Tuesday, and you allow him to take the test next Thursday, you must allow all students to take the test next Thursday. Likewise, if a student has struggled and for some reason you allow a "makeup test" in exchange for their lowest test score, this opportunity should be available for all students. While there are indeed times when that may occur (as mentioned earlier in Test Analysis), never single out one student to repeat a test to better their grade without offering it to the whole class for the same reason.

Sometimes grades are based on points; sometimes points are given but do not relate to grades. For example, based on the assignment (such as a debate, presentation, or activity), assessments may not be for points, but rather for feedback. As their mentor, your job is to guide them in their quest for knowledge and to be able to articulate their knowledge. Students may be sharing their perception or opinion or may even be presenting varying sides of a controversial issue. Perhaps they are new to the college setting and are beginning to perform literature reviews but are still a novice in defending their point of view. These situations require professional responses, constructive feedback, and an eye for where and when to introject advice. While a grade would certainly evoke a response, it is not appropriate, as the student is clearly working in the right direction. However, they need molding and guidance; your leadership style can instill this. These are great opportunities to speak one-to-one with students without any pretense or agenda. Simply being open to where they need help and how you can guide them to do the assignment better can involve trust, confidence, and self-efficacy in the student; it can also increase motivation as these other areas improve. Students often appreciate a chance to speak with their faculty without worrying about grading or the "rules" of engagement. If it is not readily or frequently available in the syllabus, allow opportunities whereby students can present their knowledge with little fear of rejection or a grade.

Formative Assessments

Official assessments are broken into formative and summative assessments. Formative assessments indicate that, as you are forming the pathway for the student's learning the material along the way, you're offering feedback. Formative assessments are ongoing, require continuous information, and may or may not have points associated with this feedback. As mentioned earlier, sometimes the feedback is more important than the grade. Summative assessment implies that you provide feedback as a summary or at the end of the course. Assessment can be as a grade or based on a rubric, test, or other assignment.

Formative assessments are often more "unofficial" and can be done impromptu. They can be a form of checks and balances to ensure the faculty member is on the right path in the instruction. It confirms that faculty are using best practices and are meeting the needs of the students. It also allows faculty to realign their focus if indeed they have gone off course. Formative assessments can be integrated fairly easily or can be a more formal evaluation. At any time when students have the chance to offer comments, render their opinion, or provide some sort of evaluation, it could be that formative assessments are occurring. Faculty should allow ample opportunities for this to occur but without judgment. Although we want to allow students to speak freely, it is not a faculty-bashing game show. Students must keep in mind the objectives, the rubric, and their roles in their own education.

Feedback Along the Way

It never hurts to ask: "How am I doing?" "Does this make sense?" or, "Are you learning?" Although you may not actually say those sentences, you may wonder if your many hours of lectures and activities are getting through. When you look at the sea of students and wonder if they are honestly listening, you could use a few interjections to check in. Sometimes it is as simple as "Is this dry material?" or "I realize this may seem boring now, but wait until we talk about (related cool topic)." You may find some students perking up and offering answers, or you may have another opportunity to readjust. Along the way it is helpful to ask such questions, but you can also ask at the end of the day. Using critical thinking questions such as "What did you learn today?" "What did you most understand?" "What is still fuzzy or muddy?" "Name three things you know now that you didn't know at the start of this class." "Name three things you liked (and didn't care for)." "What did you think about class today?" These questions allow students to speak freely and offer feedback without fear of any retaliation or consequence. It also allows them to clarify and give you some good pointers. Never be embarrassed to receive such (great) feedback—this is what you really are looking for: did I actually hit my target?

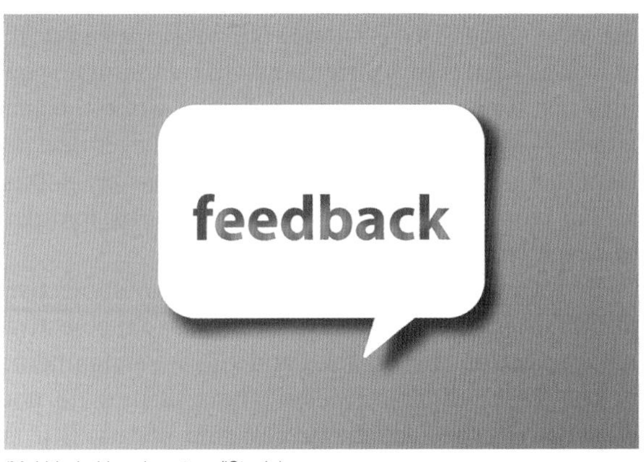

(Makhbubakhon Ismatova/iStock.)

Summative Assessments

Unlike the casual and informative sense that formative assessments have, summative assessments are very formal. They are often in the form of tests, final projects, grades and have strict rubrics. They have been formulated by other departments or committees to ensure there are reliability and validity studies to support the results. They have been tested and retested to offer the most unbiased outcome in which students could receive a grade. Whether conducted in a computer-based test, whereby results are tallied immediately, or a similar setting whereby results are tallied by a computer or faculty member, there is little leniency in the evaluation. Such information is helpful to the faculty as it puts the student and their results against other like-minded students, whether within the institution and/or against the nation or the world. If the national average is to perform 90% on an exam and your students perform at 70%, they clearly are missing some key points. It can be helpful for you as faculty to review the material to see where they missed key points. If you get the chance to redirect students before the end of the course, it helps the current students to be successful. If not, it helps the next group to be successful. This also implies that we are perpetuating best practices, as we are continuously improving.

Consider this example of a class on pharmacology. As part of your class, you review each classification and drugs within the classification, you review side effects and other important information. You engage the students with class activities, games, making their drug cards, etc. Despite all of this, one student is struggling with how drugs are classified; they have difficulty with understanding and conceptualizing this categorization and cannot grasp how to organize drugs. Your formative assessments would include the feedback you provide along the way, helping them categorize their drugs, providing flash cards, and having a peer mentor them. You do a weekly check in meeting to review their progress; you confirm what they are understanding and where they are improving, and areas they have not grasped. These formative assessments continuously guide the student toward their goal of learning the proper classifications. While these meetings are helpful, the student scores poorly on the final exam—the summative assessment. Neither you nor the student did anything wrong. It could be that in small doses the student was able to grasp basic concepts but could not pull them together in the end. Perhaps they were unable to see the bigger picture. The important point is that you gave feedback along the way, checking in for understanding and redirecting the student as often as necessary. Your formative assessments were spot on; if indeed all of the other students were able to pass the final with a 75% or higher, your summative assessment was also spot on.

Let's add a twist. Perhaps more than one student is struggling, and you have multiple tutoring sessions with the students. They do not understand or conceptualize drug classifications. In fact, they are so frustrated they are getting ready to drop the course. You chalk it up to a language barrier and tell them to just read the material more or watch some YouTube videos. In the end, they fail the final exam; in fact, they fail every test in the course. You aren't concerned because 25% of the class passed and you feel you did a good job. While you may have done a "good job" (whatever that means to you), your students did not receive the best instruction or learning opportunity. Ineffective formative assessments and lack of test analysis could have contributed to a large portion of the class failing. While there could be a language barrier (indeed pharmacology has its own language!), there needed to be more appropriate interventions. This is not to say you must do all the tutoring or provide all of the feedback; that can get overwhelming pretty quickly. Perhaps someone else on your team is good with pharmacology or can explain classifications a bit easier? If not, referring students to YouTube videos and other online tutorials could be appropriate, if you circle back and check in. These interventions are effective tools, but students still need you, as the one guiding the learning, to assess whether they are improving the learning.

Perhaps, in this same scenario, you claim that you have a full schedule and don't have more time for tutoring, but you will offer specific websites and other resources that can help explain these complicated concepts. Those who are struggling are put into two groups. You assign activities/websites to one small group of students and let them know you

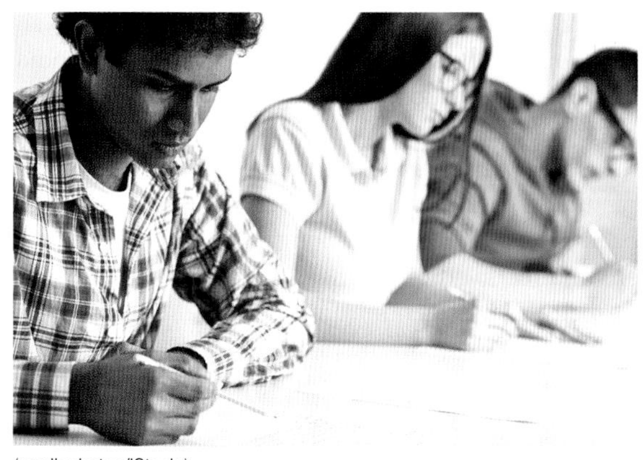
(mediaphotos/iStock.)

will reassess their understanding in 4 days. In the meantime, those who are grasping the material are asked to peer mentor the other small group who are struggling. In 4 days, you check in with each group to determine the effectiveness of your interventions: self-study versus peer mentoring. If both groups are improving, you may want to switch to ensure all students have both resources: websites, activities, and peer mentoring. If only one group is improving—see what is working. Maybe the peer mentoring group is too social, and they aren't focusing on the work. Perhaps the websites are too advanced and cannot assist an already confused student. Your evaluation of the effectiveness of these interventions is the formative assessment, even though you did not do the intervention yourself.

Total Derailment?

The art of teaching is not without frustrating moments; you may find that even with careful interventions students are simply not performing well on the test and are at risk for not passing the course. You may want to take a step back and consider a few other aspects:

- Has this course been taught before? If so, what was the pass rate?
- Who taught this course previously? Are they available to share best practices? What worked for them?
- What does your institution think about so many students struggling? If it is a prerequisite course, it may be designed to discern which students could handle the rigor of the core curriculum.
- Have you done ample test analysis? Are you covering the material in accordance with the objectives? If so, are the objectives and tests in alignment?
- If all else fails, speak with your manager and determine what you should do. Don't consider this your problem to handle without additional information or possible other interventions.

There are times when the curriculum has not been reviewed recently, and the objectives and tests may not be in alignment. While you are not responsible for the total overhaul of the course, you may have to interject other forms of assessments to determine whether students have grasped the material. Every now and then these assessments can replace a low scoring test or can be added to the average. Be an advocate for your students; if the tests are outdated or if students are being asked questions on the test you were not responsible for covering based on the lesson plan, see what else can be offered. Are there other tests you may use or other forms of assessments just as a presentation or paper? Perhaps they can do a video or infomercial (perfect for a pharmacology class!). Can you edit the tests and remove questions that are not pertinent? Can you drop the lowest test score and average the rest? Being creative and using your own critical thinking skills can be helpful for students who *do* know the material, but the assessment is not revealing it. Remember, whatever you do for one you must do for all. You cannot simply offer additional forms of assessment to a small group of students scoring poorly on a test or offer to drop their lowest score. Even if a student is getting an "A" in the course they deserve the same opportunity to raise their grade as the student receiving a "D."

Other Assessments

While tests, quizzes, and exams are the most prevalent form of summative assessments, other forms of assessments can be just as effective in determining whether the student learned the material based on the outcomes. This approach is often helpful to share with students, especially those who have test anxiety. If they hear the word "test" and get so nervous they forget their name, they may need help in decreasing that anxiety and reinforcing their learning. Having a practice round, quasi tests (not for points), presentations, pop tests, and open book quizzes can reinforce their learning so that they get used to recalling the material, applying it, and are better able to integrate it when a test question appears. Students need a neutral opportunity to reveal (or not) their learning, in addition to the assignments (e.g., exams) that are graded. These opportunities also allow the student to increase their confidence and self-efficacy, thereby increasing their opportunity to be successful on the summative assessments. Using Bloom's taxonomy will guide you as you provide these opportunities and facilitate a less stressed student when it is finals week.

Finals Week

In addition to the testing environment, faculty must be cognizant of the tests scheduled during the week or even the day. While you may not know every other professor's exam schedule, you do know your own. Keep exams days lighter if you must schedule other activities. Realize that most students feel brain-dead after an exam, so enter the next course material lightly. Perhaps start off with engagement activities, a light review of the material, and play a few games or nonthreatening exercises so students can feel positive. If the exam was a difficult one or covered difficult material, students may feel deflated and not interested in learning. They may also not be able to focus until they see their grades from the exam or the course. Make sure you reveal at what time grades will be posted and keep them focused on where you are now in their current class until that time. You may also want to reassure them of best-case scenarios—keep the energy positive.

While many students perform better earlier in the morning, consider what they did last night. Did they work all night on a paper you assigned to be due before their final exam? Are they still grasping the last lecture from yesterday to add to their understanding for today's exam? Did they leave the lecture yesterday confused, disjointed, or with more questions than answers? If you need time to recap a few minor items, be very sure to not add to their confusion. Also remind students that "studying" or "brain cramming" right before a test will not help them score better, as "brain purge" is often the least effective means to be successful on an exam. If your institution allows it, plan a fun activity after the exam, such as a potluck, an outside game (not material related), or a field trip. These activities can reduce your students' anxiety and transition them to the next lecture topic.

Surveys

Ongoing surveys can be an easy way to check in with your students to ensure they are on task. This can be created through a free website (such as Survey Monkey) or, if it was a simple question, you could use voting buttons in Outlook. You can do a quick pencil and paper survey or even a focused group survey. Whatever you choose to use, consider a few important pieces: it should be anonymous to allow students to speak freely, there can be no retaliation based on their comments, there is no incentive for completing the survey, and answers are confidential (with respect to the institution's policy). Surveys can be time consuming to create but can also be used more than once, even within each class.

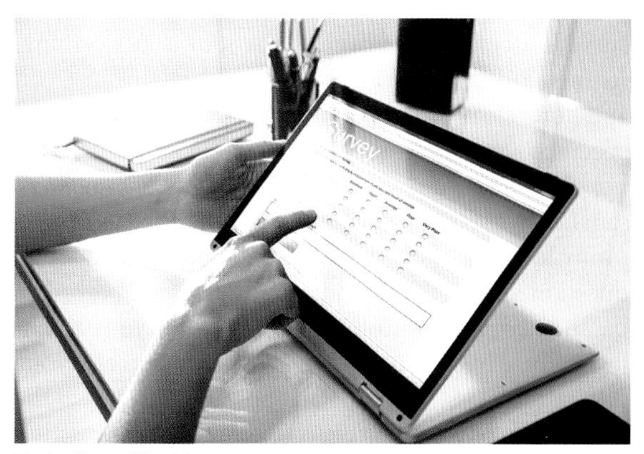

(AndreyPopov/iStock.)

In addition to your own surveys, your institution may use surveys for students, faculty, and outside facilities (such as a clinical or externship site). This feedback provides a more complete picture of the student's learning opportunity and the resources provided to facilitate this learning. If surveys are sent to students to evaluate the course and the faculty, those comments or scores may also be part of the faculty's evaluation. Likewise, if students and faculty can evaluate the clinical or externship sites, this information is used at advisory board meetings to ensure students are receiving adequate learning off site. Students often are asked to evaluate their overall experience, including their experience of other departments. Are there ample places for them to work on a computer, print their papers, or get support if they have information technology (IT) issues? Did the admissions team inform them of the expectations for the program accurately? Are there other resources the student needed to be successful that may have been advertised but were not available? Though these are campus-driven improvements, it is good to be aware of any obstacle that impedes your students' ability to be successful. If they were planning on using a computer in the library to do their work and there are not enough computers or the library is closed on weekends, the student now has additional challenges that were not present when they enrolled.

Satisfaction

Many institutions employ outside companies (or internal departments) to conduct satisfaction surveys; these surveys ascertain how well the school is performing. As mentioned, many areas are included, not just you and your class. However, your surveys can be related specifically to how well you explained the material, how available you were, and whether students were satisfied with your teaching. Often there is an opportunity for the student to make comments related to the question and elaborate more fully. These surveys can be an effective tool to look objectively at your teaching style. While faculty often feel good when everyone passes the class, it is not an indication whether the teaching style was effective or the methods of instruction worked.

Satisfaction surveys should provide objective and constructive remarks from students. However, as mentioned, it should not be taken personally if there are negative comments. Some students need a space to voice their concern, regardless of whether it is constructive or simply a sounding board. However, as you go through the comments, see if there is a common denominator. Perhaps it seemed that you were always rushed or that you were running late. Maybe you were extremely approachable in class, but your office hours were not conducive to a student's needs. Students may have felt that they enjoyed your class, but they did not learn as much as they had hoped. These comments require a moment of reflection, as they have some very good points. Although you may not know which class or course offered these comments, consider it an ongoing improvement plan. As you review each comment, check in with yourself and determine what you can do differently next class to address these issues, or if you have changed a few things, were the changes in the "right" direction.

End of the Course

Often these evaluations come at the end of the course, like a summative assessment for you and your class. It is important to use this information (whenever you received it) to reflect and re-evaluate your teaching methods. However, don't wait for this survey to do some reflecting. Just as students perform ongoing assessments, you should be evaluating your own best practices, what has worked, and what you need to tweak. You will know better than anyone what has worked, what needs help, and where you need to employ different tactics for the next course. As you have gone (or go) through your course, hopefully you have been taking notes or will take notes. Your "notes to self" will be extremely helpful to ensure you have less stress and more insight in your next class/course. Just as students are continuously improving, so are faculty.

What to Do With Assessment Results

Before you go out and buy a pint of your favorite ice cream to help you digest the student satisfaction survey results, keep in mind that everyone is entitled to their opinion, and everyone has a different perception. If you keep this in mind, you can look at results a bit more objectively. Consider a food analogy: let's equate your course to preparing hamburgers for your students. Although there are a variety of ways to serve hamburgers, you chose to go with traditional. You prepare the meat with 85% lean beef, add salt and pepper (perhaps some Worcestershire and garlic), and grill it to medium perfection; you serve it with condiments (mayo and mustard, pickles, lettuce, ketchup, onions, and Heinz 57). Though you feel that you did a great job with hamburgers, some people prefer turkey burgers, some prefer cheeseburgers, some like ground sirloin, others enjoy sautéed mushrooms and onions, and still others are vegetarians. Even with the vegetarians there are certain brands that vegetarians prefer, such as Boca Burgers, Morningstar, Beyond Meat, and Garden Burgers. Your survey results may indicate your students did not like your traditional burger, because you did not introduce or include all previous seven options. Perhaps the expectation from your students was that they would have a sample of every kind of burger there is, and thus they are disappointed.

This analogy goes back to knowing your audience. In the first class, orientation, or initial interview, did you get a chance to determine their expectations? If not, you may find out in retrospect. Now armed with this knowledge, you can start each new class with the fact that this class will only cover the classic hamburger – not vegetarian burgers, cheeseburgers, or any other variation, but your basic and simple generic hamburger. While you hope that they will learn a variety of ways to prepare this classic burger, it is still simply a basic burger.

Although this analogy seems simplistic, it still reviews some fundamental principles. Knowing your audience; thinking about what expectations students have prior to class; being aware of what else they may want or feel they need and reviewing what relates to the course. If students expect you to discuss hot dogs in your course, and mark you less in points because you didn't, don't feel incompetent. Hot dogs are nowhere near hamburgers, except in common comfort foods at a barbeque. If, however, they are concerned about your ability to know the difference between a hamburger and a fish burger, perhaps that favorite ice cream is needed. All joking aside, keep in mind what the survey results rate and whether or not it applies to you. Be honest, objective, and professional in your review; don't take it personally but do take it with some incentive to improve. Just as with your course, you want to focus on *your* best practices and make the next course better. Not that you come out being liked by all students, but that you are effective in helping students reach their goals in education.

Student's Self-assessments

As much as we focus on assessments of student performance and faculty surveys, we must also hold students accountable for their own assessments. Students should be performing ongoing self-evaluations of their learning. They should know what else they need and where to obtain it in their quest to understand the material. In reviewing their syllabus and expectations, students should be aware of due dates, assignment criteria, rubrics, and exams. If they have questions, they should ask. If they do not understand or need further clarification, they should seek out the faculty during office hours (which is why they are on the syllabus). In short, as we have focused on student-centered learning, with the student guiding their quest, we should expect students to know when they are off course. In an ideal world, we should. However, chances are, with few exceptions, we won't. Few students will be so proactive and seek you out, know what they need, and seek your guidance in how to get there. However, many others won't have a clue and need more direction from you.

This is not to say you cannot teach a student to learn how to self-assess or to seek guidance in their inefficient areas. Obviously, you can direct such willing students if they are doing the work and not relying on you to constantly direct them. As you remind them of what their course is, also remind them of how they will identify *how* the objectives will be met. This may prompt them to review what the objectives are or how they will arrive at the stated objectives. The important part is that active learning is taking place, with the emphasis on *active*.

Practice Round

Let's imagine you are teaching a class on surgical tools. We shall identify the goals, objectives and outcomes, create a rubric, identify appropriate tests/assessments, using both formative and summative assessments.

Goals, objectives, and outcomes. The surgical class is an 8-week course to help students identify basic surgical tools used in the operating room (OR) at the local community hospital. Tools used are for adult medical patients only, not obstetrics (OB), pediatrics, or any specialty surgery. At the completion of this class, students will correctly identify the 50 primary tools used in the OR. They will demonstrate proper techniques in a sterile field, an autoclave, and in inventory. The goal is to prepare students for a career in health care. The objective is that students learn the primary tools used in the OR for general adult medical surgical patients. The outcome is that the students will correctly identify the 50 tools and demonstrate knowledge of a sterile field, perform a written test on the appropriate use of tools, and appropriately identify which tools should be in the inventory for basic procedures.

Create a rubric. When students are asked to identify the 50 tools used in common medical procedures, the following rubric will be used. Total points = 30 points. Students can repeat this exercise only once, after a 2-hour remediation in between. If the students cannot perform the minimum standard (poor), they will fail each category and score a zero. The passing score needed is 50% or 15/30 points (*Table 7.1*).

Tests/assessments. In addition to the verbal demonstration, students must align each tool in the respective space as was set up for various procedures. Students will be given 15 minutes to set up their tools in accordance with the procedure. After setting up the tools in their designated space, students will be asked once if they have any changes. Total set up must be completed within 20 minutes in preparation for the procedure. This demonstration is worth 50 points and is pass/fail. Students can remediate twice and repeat the demonstration in order to achieve a passing score. A final exam worth 100 points will be given at the completion of the course. This exam is open book and must be conducted during the class time (2 hours). There is no makeup test; failure to complete this exam on the class day or within the 2-hour period will result in a zero.

Formative assessments. Six lab periods are given in order to provide practice time. During these times, the lab instructor will review the tools, how to pronounce them, spell them, and what they are used for. Students are encouraged to use this time as frequently as possible. (While this is on your syllabus, you will check in with the lab instructor to ensure students are utilizing the lab time asking questions and have improved in their pronunciation. You may even use some class time in addition to lab time to ask students to do an inventory of the tools used in common surgical procedures, play games on how to pronounce the names of common tools, and do a matching exercise to ascertain they have learned what tools are used in various medical procedures. Students who are unable to complete these exercises may need additional tutoring by you, the lab instructor, or more time to review the material outside of class.)

Summative assessments. The final exam comprises four components: naming the tools, identifying what they are used for, how to set up the procedure or surgery, and what other tools may be used in addition. The final exam is worth

TABLE 7.1 Sample Rubric for Surgical Tools

	Excellent = 10 Points	Good = 8 Points	Fair = 5 Points	Poor = 3 Points
Identify tools	Can identify at least 40 tools	Can identify at least 30 tools	Can identify at least 25 tools	Can identify at least 10 tools
Pronunciation of tools	Of the tools identified, can properly pronounce at least 30 of the 40 tools	Of the tools identified, can properly pronounce at least 20 of the 30 tools	Of the tools identified, can properly pronounce at least 15 of the 25 tools	Of the tools identified, can properly pronounce at least five of the 10 tools
Tool usage	Of the tools identified, can correctly state what the tool is used for in at least 30 of the 40 tools	Of the tools identified, can correctly state what the tool is used for in at least 20 of the 30 tools	Of the tools identified, can correctly state what the tool is used for in at least 15 of the 25 tools	Of the tools identified, can correctly state what the tool is used for in at least five of the 10 tools

100 points and is given during class. Two hours is allotted for the exam, which is open book. Personal notes are allowed, but peer assistance is not. Any student caught cheating, discussing answers, talking to peers, or sharing notes will be given a zero. (This is on your syllabus, is explained to students in detail at the beginning of class, and is shared toward the time for the final. Nothing is a surprise; students should know fully what is expected.)

Conclusion

In this sample exercise, it was clear what students were expected to know, how they could get assistance, how they would be graded, what alternative they had for remediation, and how many points each evaluation was worth for the verbal demonstration and the final. The student who comes to you wondering why they received only 13 points on the verbal demonstration can easily be responded to. Even though they were proud of the fact they could identify 20 tools and could pronounce and identify usage on 15 tools, according to the rubric, they earned only 13 points. In review of their remediation, you noted that they never went to the lab (the instructor has no attendance record of them being present for remediation or practice) and they were never present during your review of tools in class. Unfortunately, they forgot their book on the final day and were unable to review it for the final exam. They spent most of the 2 hours worried about their book and did not answer all the questions within the allotted timeframe. The student failed the course with 60%. Few arguments can defend their lack of involvement or preparation for the assessments. Their counterpart, however, was present for every lab, was able to identify 40 tools, including correct pronunciation, inventory, and usage. This student reviewed the material and brought their book for the final with highlighted key terms. This student was able to complete the answers in the 2-hour period and passed the course with a 95%.

Journal: Self-reflection

1 Before doing a practice assessment on your own, describe your feelings and comfort level with assessments in general.

a. Describe your comfort level with giving constructive/negative feedback:

____

____

____

b. Share your ability to create rubrics—are you clear on how to create or use one?

____

____

____

c. What is your experience in designing goals, objectives, and creating outcomes? If you have no experience, what is your confidence level in each of these? Do you know the difference between them?

____

____

____

____

____

____

Be sure to review the above with your manager or peer mentor to ensure you have a clear understanding of these terms and their usage.

2 Considering the course(s) you will be teaching, what are the things you will want to assess (in addition to the material)? List five things you want to assess:

a. ______
b. ______
c. ______
d. ______
e. ______

3 How will you assess these things? List one way you will assess each item listed in #2.

a. ______
b. ______
c. ______
d. ______
e. ______

4 Ongoing feedback is important to ensure you and your students are on the right trajectory. List three ways you will use this style of assessment in your class.

______
______
______
______
______
______

5 Pretend that you are teaching your course tomorrow. While you may (or may not) be ready, you must gather what you have and at least have a lesson plan for the week, including a syllabus, homework, class activities, and two assessments. Each work/test/assessment must have a rubric. Using this as the start, create the following: the homework, class activities, two assessments, and rubric. This is just for *this* week.

Class subject (be specific): ______
Objective: ______
Goal(s): ______
Outcome: ______

Briefly describe your lesson plan for the week:

______
______
______
______
______
______
______
______
______

Homework for this week (or the weekend):

Rubric for homework assignment: (draw a table if desired)

Class activities for the week (list three in-class activities):

Rubric for each class activity: (draw a table if desired)

#1 Assessment: what form of assessment will you use? What are you measuring?

Rubric for #1 Assessment: (draw a table if desired)

#2 Assessment: what form of assessment will you use? What are you measuring?

Rubric for #2 Assessment: (draw a table if desired)

6 The testing environment is crucial.

a. How will you ensure that students are able to maintain test integrity as well as their own accountability during exams?

b. How will you create a positive testing environment? (List two things you will do.)

7 In your own words, describe the formative and summative assessment that you will be using for your course.

a. Formative assessments:

b. Summative assessments:

8 Consider that you have a task or skill that students must do in your class. This can be a related skill in your curriculum or even a soft skill. If you are teaching a course that does not require a specific skill, perhaps you assess students' abilities to follow rules, be on time, speak professionally, and work in teams. Choose one skill that you will assess.

a. What is this skill?

b. How will students demonstrate they know this skill?

c. How will you assess that they have met the requirements for this skill?

d. Create a checklist for this skill: (draw a table if desired)

9 Self-assessments are a part of every student and faculty member's ongoing improvement. Name three things that you will instill in your students to provide ongoing self-evaluation and improvement.

10 Name three things that *you* will do to provide your own ongoing self-evaluation and improvement.

All great achievements require time.
Maya Angelou

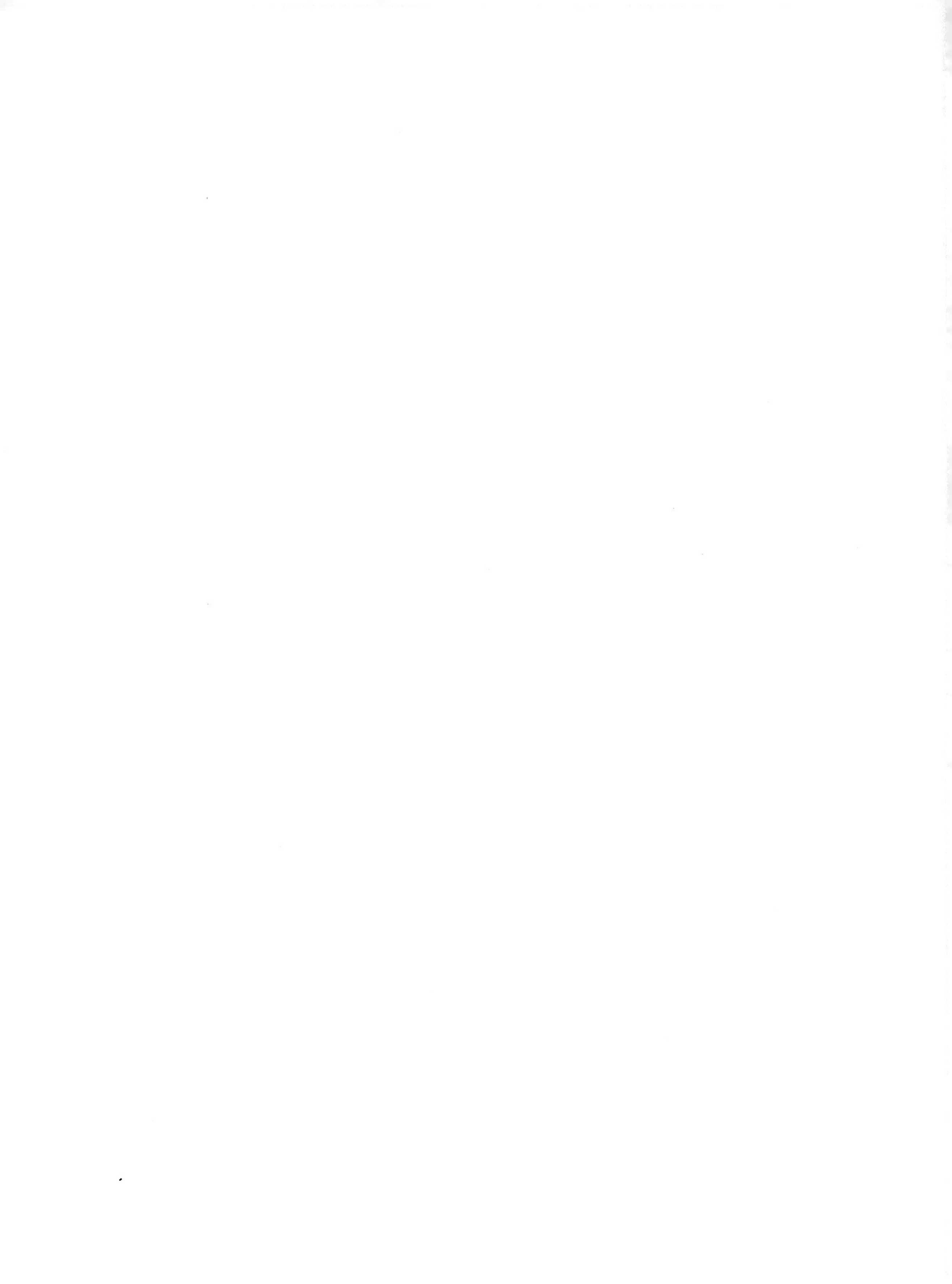

Chapter 8

Decreasing the Generational Gap

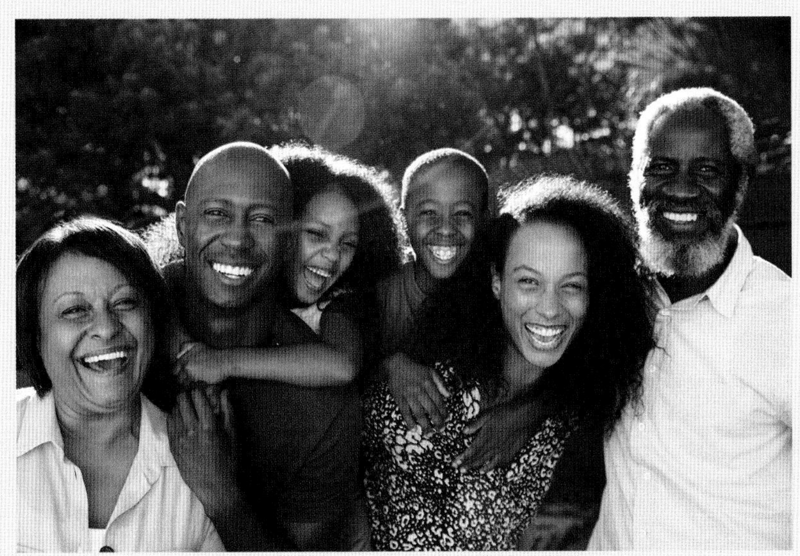

(monkeybusinessimages/iStock.)

As we consider the many attributes that we as faculty have, and that our students have, there may be some things we have in common; there may also be great differences. Although we have focused on how differences help us understand other perspectives and support diversity, we also need to better understand where these differences come from. Each perspective is compiled from a variety of influences, as mentioned in our previous chapters. This chapter, however, will focus specifically on where those perspectives come from; primarily, based on each generation. Most faculty are not in the same generation as those that they teach; in fact, one of the obstacles you must overcome is to teach to an older or younger generation than your own. It is helpful to see what global perspective these generations have in order to determine where there are potential conflicts, needs, similarities, and strengths.

My Generation

One of the most influential perspectives (other than one's culture) is societal, based on the society we lived in during our upbringing years. This perspective provides the basis for "classifying" a generation, or when considering what generation you are from. Although some websites want to pigeon-hole generations based on when you were born, most research supports the fact that generation is based on your perspective—the events you recall and what was influential to you regarding education, politics, technology, and the economy. It also is based on geography, as some countries may have less influence of these traits than others. Though *Table 8.1* is not an absolute (as no such chart exists), it does offer the common references for the generations living during 2020.

In reviewing these generations, you can see how some of these attributes can be a problem in the

TABLE 8.1 Generations

Generation	Range of Birth Year	Memorable Moments	Attributes
Silent Generation	1925–1945	Invention of wireless radios Suffered the Great Depression Saw the rise in motor vehicles, aircrafts, and transportation	Very patriotic Employer takes care of you, thus very loyal to a job
Baby Boomers	1946–1964	Post-WWII and post-Vietnam War Invention of TV, cassettes, etc. "Sexual revolution" hippies Rise in women in the workforce	Brand loyal Focus is on going up the corporate ladder
Gen X	1965–1976	Post-Cold War Latchkey kids MTV *Challenger* explodes Crash of the stock market IBM PC, Walkman, VCR Rise in student debt	Conspiracy theorists Focus is on self-improvement
Millennials (Gen Y)	1977–1995	Internet, Netflix, increase in social media, email, reality TV 9/11 School shootings	Focus is on friends, less loyalty to business employer as you need to gain more experiences
Gen Z (iGen or Centennials)	1996–present	Grew up with all of the current technology, including Google, Twitter, etc. Have never seen major war Emergence of e-learning	Focus is on a worldly environment, want responses quickly and eco-friendly

classroom. For example, a Millennial (Marlice) is working with a Baby Boomer (Bob) on a group project; Marlice says she will text Bob and send a link to the website they need to refer to. Bob is embarrassed and says he doesn't know how to pull up a link, or really even how to text. Marlice is wondering how anyone could not understand how to use a smartphone to text! Bob admits that he has little experience with technology; Marlice shares she has little patience and no reference point. How can these two students work on a project together?

As their teacher, you must have both the patience and foresight before assigning these two to a group; you must let them know that they may have to overcome obstacles. Indeed, we will all have to work with people who know more or know less than we do; skills aside, we must still get the job done. Marlice's job will require patience when working with customers, patients/clients, or even other employees. The soft skills of professionalism, courtesy, and providing the time needed to review how to look up the link on a smartphone can be helpful in a variety of settings. Likewise, you may approach Bob and see what he *does* know about his smartphone. Perhaps he just switched from an Android to an iPhone; maybe he never really got a good orientation on how to use the features. Marlice can also show Bob how to send this information from his phone to his computer, if Bob is more comfortable looking things up on his laptop instead of the small screen on a phone. Whatever the obstacle, both students must understand they are seeing the work from different perspectives, and each person has something to offer.

On the flip side, Marlice gets frustrated easily and often loses focus from one project to the next. She is currently scoring low on her tests and forgets to submit her homework. Bob is perplexed how anyone could forget to turn in an assignment, as he religiously submits his work early and performs very well on the tests. As a Baby Boomer, he values authority and has been able to follow along with each lecture. Bob thinks Marlice acts like his grandson who has been diagnosed with attention deficit hyperactivity disorder (ADHD), but realizes he cannot ask her if she has a diagnosis. He does ask if she would like some helpful hints on how to perform better on tests, and if he can work with her on a schedule so she can remember to submit (and complete) her assignments. While this interaction may come out naturally from one caring student to another, you may also have to suggest such ideas or use your intuition to nudge the conversation. "Hey Bob, I see that you have been doing a great job with submitting all of your homework on time. I sincerely appreciate this—what's your secret?" "Marlice, you have shared with me that sometimes you get frustrated. I think Bob has done some work with other students who get frustrated—do you mind if he shares some key points that have helped? Maybe they can help you—maybe not, but it might be worth a try!"

In addition to understanding the similarities and differences between generations it is also important to note what they value. The older generations (Silent Generation and Baby Boomers) have considerable loyalty to their employers, businesses, and service industries. In fact, they know more about customer service than other generations (Gen Xers do too). This can be a great discussion in a class of Millennials who wants to focus on the use of technology and how much easier it makes life. However, Millennials often fail to understand how technology can estrange them from their customers or clients. For example, older generations focused a great deal on customer service, such as full-service gas stations (you mean they checked your oil, too?), travel agencies (long before Kayak, Travelocity, and Expedia), and rewarded loyalty (such as S&H Green Stamps, which later would be redeemed for something out of their catalog). They spend time talking with the grocery clerk or waitress, ensure they always leave a tip, and are more apt to say hello to a passerby. They value human interaction and aren't as rushed to get through the day. This is not because they are ready for retirement, necessarily, but because they appreciate a non–technology-based world. They are not into Siri or Alexa, but rather communicating with another fellow human being.

Millennials value human beings, but on a more global basis. They use the advancement of technology to facilitate this communication, such as the Internet, emails, and social media. This generation does not understand the concept of boundaries related to staying in one country (they often have traveled to more countries than their ancestors), and they may appear to be less patriotic. They are often considered the "me" generation, as they focus on how any information will improve their life, livelihood, or current status. They don't have much loyalty to just one business as they see opportunities on a worldly level; they seek answers from this universal perspective to help them gain better insight.

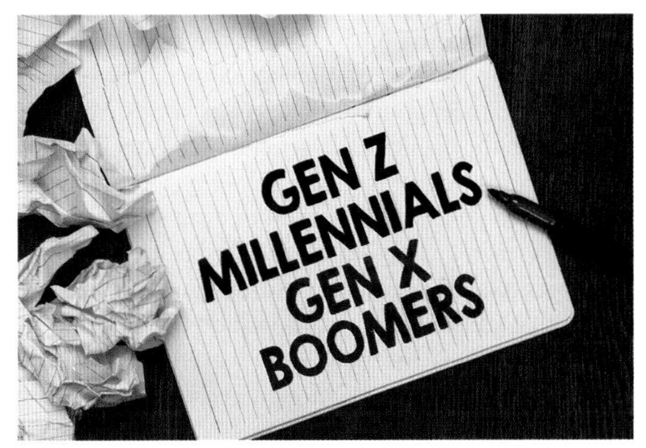

(Artur/iStock.)

Gen Xers value both people and technology and are sandwiched in between these two generations, which can make it both an asset and a disadvantage. This generation can attest to the discovery of new technology and are often savvy with such technology; however, they are often not experts (unless they studied this field). While they may be able to help Bob, Marlice can still surpass the Gen Xer with her knowledge and speed. Gen Xers often tend to be perfectionist, as much as they are conspiracy theorists (hence the need for self-reliance). Gen Xers and Baby Boomers value education and respect authority; they could be good examples of leadership in a very structured class. However, they can be insulted if students are allowed to speak out of turn, create their own assignments and due dates, and may struggle with this "free form" approach to education. Both Millennials and Gen Zers will be the ones who expect technology, negotiable rules, and could lead a small group if it meant using social media and the Internet to find answers.

Though there are many differences between generations, there are also many similarities. Each generation feels that other generations don't understand them, and they wonder what's happening with these other generations. They joke about what life was like when they were younger (except the youngest—Gen Z), and how current generations wouldn't have a clue. They often see all people through the lens of their own generation and make judgments accordingly. Yet each generation has had an emergence of something that impacted our world and made history, whether it was a war, TV, the Internet, or social media. They wonder how the earlier generations could get by without new inventions and believe their generation has made the best contribution to society. Each generation has shaped history with their music, their political stands, and a next wave of ____ (fill in the blank). Each generation has their group of rebels, kids who dress differently (e.g., Gothic), who are proud to go against the grain or against the crowd. However, each generation also looks back on simpler times, reflects on what life could be like if not for the things that cause conflict. Old fashions come back in style, "vintage" is the new "cool"; even slang words and phrases get repeated (though perhaps not "gnarly dude!"). While many generations think they want world peace, a world without wars, and everybody to get along, not everyone strives for this goal. As a group of like-minded individuals, a generation identifies itself with how it views the world around them and how they interact with this world. It gleans from what the generations before them have done but doesn't necessarily agree on how to improve society or the world we now live in. Sometimes, current generations blame previous generations and want to omit or change the past. When using class discussions as an opportunity to review, compare, or contrast history and world events, be cautious if students want to complain about the "sins of their fathers." If we negate history, we often will repeat it as we never learned from our mistakes. Help students see why *that* generation had to do what they did during that timeframe. Acknowledge that hindsight is 20/20 and that as we move forward, we hope to improve our circumstances (if not our world) by making incremental changes or at least increasing our awareness. No generation has perfected anything; we are all a work in progress. The next generation will undoubtedly criticize this generation, and the cycle continues.

Ages

Though it may seem that generations equate to ages, there are differences as the broad age range in the generation classification lends itself to such a gap. Consider an older Millennial (born in 1977) and a younger Gen Z (born in 2002); these two students have a 25-year difference, despite the fact that they are only one generation apart. Moreover, the Millennial could be the parental age of the Gen Z student. In another example, a student could have a parent within their own generation (if the parent bore children at a young age). A 16-year-old girl, born in 1977, gives birth to a child born in 1993—both are Millennials, born in the same generation. This in and of itself offers challenges as the closer the generation, the more friction. There is research which supports the notion that the further apart generations are, the better the relationship is. Other research suggests that attributes within a generation repeat themselves after one or two cycles, so a Baby Boomer and a Millennial may have similar attributes or viewpoints as the Baby Boomer and Gen Xer. This could be why older grandparents and their younger grandchildren often have a closer relationship than the parent and child (of course, it could also have something to do with how much grandparents spoil their grandchildren!).

Age also has to do with maturity. Just because someone is 18 years old does not mean they are immature any more than being 30 years old means they are mature. As an instructor, it is important to ascertain who has more tendencies toward maturity, responsibilities, and accountability. It may also come down to communication and how this information is relayed to you. While one student may want to send you a Skype request after class, another may want to FaceTime at midnight (past your own bedtime). Work with what fits best in your schedule. Based on ages, some students may be in a sandwich generation (currently Gen Xers); this implies that they have children they are still raising or caring for, as well as aged parents. This added responsibility may make it difficult to prioritize educational needs with the responsibilities at home. Although it is helpful to be sympathetic, it is more important to help the student consider their own needs, self-care, and resources that will facilitate the student being successful. Many times, a student will fall victim to their circumstances and not consider themselves the priority. When this occurs, their grades may suffer, they may not be as attentive during class, and in fact may need to leave class or simply not be present. This puts the student at risk for not being successful in the class and may contribute to their stress level. If your institution offers community resources or other support services, it is best to introduce these early so the students can feel more at ease during class time.

Civility

The art of being polite, courteous, and kind may seem like a no brainer to many generations, however, our current society feels this art is waning. In order to reconnect people with this art, there are classes, requirements, and training to safeguard students. It is important to be aware of this training and count it as valuable. Just as you have come to realize "common sense" may not be so common, civility is not part of every person's repertoire of behavior. It could be due to their upbringing, their desire to rebel, or simply cultural differences. While you may ask why they behave a certain way, you can also enlighten them that this behavior is considered rude or disrespectful and is not tolerated in the class or group exercises.

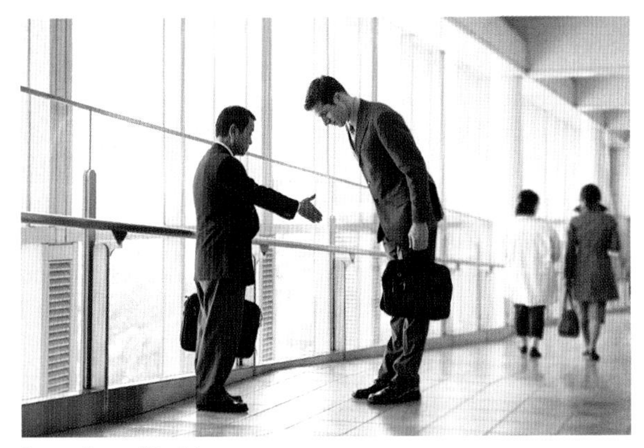

(Image Source/iStock.)

Culture

Interwoven with generations is our culture. Some cultures evolve as rapidly or as slowly as others, some do so within their region of the world. Some cultures differ based on geographical areas of the United States, while others vary based on continent. As mentioned in Chapter 2, a person from New York may not seem to have much in common with the person from Alabama. Their respective geographical cultures may influence how they speak to others, their religious affiliations, and how they view "outsiders." They may be xenophobic or may be very outgoing and open to others. The person from Alabama may have more respect for authority, may say "yes ma'am" and "no sir," especially if they are a Gen Xer or older. The person from New York may find no harm in being gregarious; they may seem very social or even more blunt than their soft-spoken Alabama counterpart. Of course, these are stereotypes, but they do illustrate how different areas within the United States can have varying cultures and how important it is to not prejudge anyone based on where they are from.

Outside the United States there are cultural regions, often based on geography. Asian countries (Japan, Thailand, China, etc.) share similar beliefs in respecting elders, honoring the family and the rules within the household, and are not typically boisterous. Filipino cultures share similar values, especially when it comes to careers. Eastern European cultures (Russian, Ukraine, Czech Republic) also have similar views on family/parenting, how to interact with others, and may appear rigid in following rules. They may seem outspoken and blunt (much like the New Yorker), but also extremely faithful to their religious beliefs. While the focus on family seems to weave between cultures, what they focus on may differ. For example, while some cultures consider it a part of their responsibility to care for a dying grandmother at all costs, others may not consider extending life a respectable option. Because they do respect their ailing grandmother, euthanasia or allowing the person to die without any intervention is a way to allow them to end their life with dignity.

World Events

As many students (and faculty) look at the actual dates of generations (see *Table 8.1*), they may not relate to that specific generation. This is especially true if the person is close on their birth date; for example, a Millennial may feel more like a Gen Xer if they were born in 1978 or 1979. The events that they recall from their childhood include watching *Dallas*, hearing the horrible story of Jim Jones' cult, and collecting Susan B. Anthony dollars. They still are wary of Bluetooth and prefer listening to their iPod. Their perspective is based on what they (and their family) were involved with. Again, some places in the United States may focus on more worldly events and others may not—this contributes to how a person connects with their generation based on events that occur worldwide and whether or not they are important. This can be a way to engage the class (or small groups) for a discussion of world events. Ask students to name the top events that have occurred during their lifetime, specifically those events that have shaped their lives—meaning it is something they will never forget. Obviously, events like 9/11 could be very meaningful; most people recall exactly where they were and what they were doing when the news came on. However, Gen Zers have no recollection of hearing this news; they have only heard it from their parents or others alive during that time period.

Current Events

In addition to the world events, current events influence a generation. As each generation interacts with today's society, they form different opinions, judgments, and use these interactions to form perceptions. Most people have heard the statement, "kids nowadays don't know about ..." or "in my day we'd never let folks get away with ..." These statements reflect the opinion one generation has on another based on current events. This can be seen with the topic of parenting, for example. If you are conducting a class on child development, you may mention that some cultures still use corporal punishment as part of their discipline. As mentioned in Chapter 3, some states allow this in the home and in schools. However, while it is not very popular nowadays, some cultures still support this to ensure children obey rules. If a student/parent says they swat their child on the bottom and put them in time out when the child misbehaves, it's not necessary to call Child Protective Services. While current standards may not reflect this as a parenting option, the student/parent's culture does. Younger parents, based on current practices, may abhor such use of force and think it unnecessary and disrespectful to the child. However, within that culture, this parenting style is supported, accepted, and in their minds, effective. On another note, younger generations may speak freely and even talk back to older generations; an act they feel no remorse for. However, the older generations may consider it rude or disrespectful. They may have a difficult time when students argue with you, the teacher (an elder who deserves respect), walk out of the room, or yell out their answers.

Point of Reference

It is important to reflect on what society allows as a "current" practice and share it with your students as a point of reference. For example, though corporal punishment is not popular with current parenting practices, there was a time when it was acceptable and would not (even by today's standards) be seen as child abuse. When a child touched something they weren't supposed to and got a swat on their hand along with a reminder to not touch the object, they often recalled that with less pain than touching a harmful object. If a parent yells at their child to get out of the road, it is far more effective than sitting them down and explaining that a car is on its way. While current parenting practice gives more focus to informing the child of best practices and asking the child if they understand, it is not necessarily appropriate when there is an emergency.

Different generations might share other practices that seemed appropriate during their time, especially as the society "norm" was different. Women, for example, did not always have the opportunity to be career minded until the late 1960s. Although there are always exceptions, society at large didn't expect a woman, if she were a mother, to work outside the home. In fact, the term "work outside of the home" wasn't prevalent before 2000. As it became more the norm for mothers to work, the expectation was that at least one parent had to work if not both. In 2018, over 70% of women with children made up the workforce; as a result, the overall national unemployment rate (for families) decreased, as one member of the household was working.

A fun exercise with your students (if you have myriad generations in your class) is to ask students to share something about the following terms or concepts.

Their answers will vary based on where they grew up, when they grew up, and the culture they are from.

- Do they refer to their evening meal as dinner or supper?
- Other than making mac and cheese, do they call it macaroni, noodles, or pasta?
- Do they know a time period before Disney?
- Do they recall black and white TV shows, even as reruns?
- Were they allowed to play outside freely or did they have scheduled play dates?
- How do they feel about cannabidiol (CBD), legalized marijuana, or using marijuana for medical reasons?
- Do they have a garbage disposal?

While some students will say "Duh, of course ...," they may be enlightened to discover not everyone has the same answer. Different responses can also trigger additional questions, especially with the garbage disposal. For example, if a student lives in the country and is on a well system, they may not have a garbage disposal. This could spark another conversation about life outside the city.

Based on your class and students' interest, you may wish to offer additional games or discussion opportunities to allow different generations to discuss their similarities and their differences as they relate to current events. Cultures who foster a closer relationship between parents and children may find the discussion easier, as Millennials can reference their parents or grandparents having the same views as the Baby Boomers and Gen Xers in the group. Students who are not close with their parents, consider themselves a free spirit, or who don't feel like they fit in may struggle with these discussions. Keep an eye on each group to ensure no one is dominating the conversation or going down too many memory lanes. Always give them a topic to reference their discussion with such as: think of one form of technology we use nowadays that you would have difficulty living without. It can be something simple like electricity, a microwave or coffee pot, a vehicle or other form of transportation, or a more current device like your phone. Allow them time to reflect, share, and report to the larger group to see what life could be like without some of more common technology advances. You can also have each generation share what skills they possess (nontechnical) that are transferable; how can being a mother equate to running a small business? How can being the bread winner help you be a better Chief Financial Officer? It will illuminate the value of even the simplest strength so that each generation, regardless of their ages, can see how they are a valuable member of today's society.

Veterans and the Military

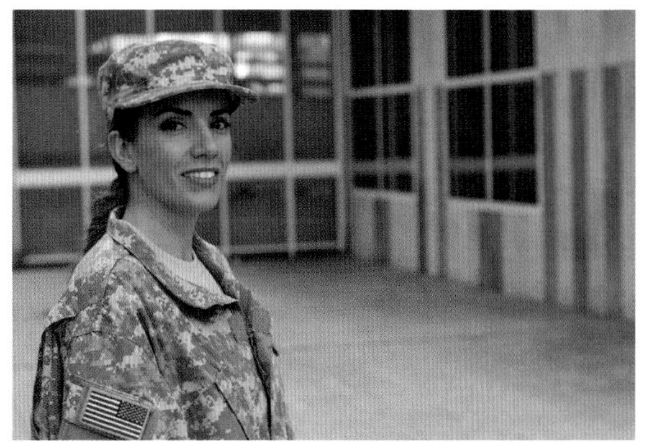

(ajr_images/iStock.)

Mixed in with the various generations are those who have served in the Armed Forces. Many military families support and encourage multiple family members to enter the military service. It is not uncommon for a family to have numerous members of the family, even several generations, serving in the Armed Forces. While older generations may have done so due to the government (draft) requirement, they either felt it was their duty and passed on this virtue to their descendants, or they appreciated the benefits of the military and wanted to see their children receive the same. While they may have served honorably, not every generation appreciated their service. Some veterans are afraid to claim their status as their generation (e.g., postwar) was not appreciative of the use of military forces to resolve conflicts in other countries.

A few terms are necessary to ensure you understand who is currently serving and who has previously served in the military. Veterans are people who have previously served in the military, regardless of the amount of time. Active duty military are people currently serving and under orders from the military to do a job. The Reserves or National Guard requires service more sporadically, such as 2 weeks a year and weekends. If one of your students is on active duty or is a Reservist, it is important to know whether they will be missing class. Military orders are not negotiable and may not allow the student to adhere to attendance policies, regardless of how it impacts the student. A 25-year-old female student may have served only 3 years in the Marines, but she is a veteran just as much as the 60-year-old who did three tours in the Middle East. Most military are amicable to their fellow military colleagues and veterans, however, never assume. Also, while many military men and women served honorably and are proud of their heritage and service, this is not always the case. Many veterans suffer from posttraumatic stress disorder (PTSD) or perhaps had a negative experience in the military. They may have been medically discharged, dishonorably discharged, or simply may not have enjoyed their tour. Always be sure to ask how their experience was in the military (if they choose to share).

God and Country

Those who have served in the military may seem more patriotic, and some may feel strongly about defending our country; however, other groups are equally as supportive of their nation. Outside of the military are service groups (such as the Lions Club), fraternity organizations (such as the Elks, Moose Lodges), and first responders (such as police and sheriff personnel, firefighters, and emergency personnel). It is important to recognize these groups and ascertain their viewpoint in addition to the veteran and military students. Do not assume that these students are any more supportive or appreciative about their service; indeed, many lives have been lost while protecting others. If appropriate, acknowledge all students for their service and for supporting and serving our community and our nation. Keep in mind that some will accept the recognition, and others may not.

In addition to the service fields, many older generations are prone to being religious, while the younger generations are often less religious but are spiritual. Older generations often went to church, the synagogue, or attended another form of worship. They usually made it part of their Saturday or Sunday, complete with a social activity afterward (e.g., coffee and donuts, a potluck, or a barbeque). Their expectation was to refer to their religious upbringing on all matters that involved their family, money, relationships, and sometimes even careers. They referenced a book, such as a *Bible*, the *Torah*, the *Qur'an*, or the *Book of Mormon*. The verses or scriptures used in these books were tools to guide one in their quest for harmony, or to follow the laws of the church. Younger generations often see their spiritual connection through involvement with others, nature, or a more worldly approach. They may consider yoga and meditation as a form of spiritual practice, may attend 12-step meetings, or may believe hiking puts them in touch with the universe. While you do not want to open a discussion with a compare/contrast on religious versus spiritual beliefs, you could open a discussion about how each practice has similarities, with a common goal of peace. Younger generations may be surprised how much they have in common with their older peers; perhaps they didn't enjoy church because it was a "have to" versus a choice. Older students may realize that their younger peers enjoy old hymnal music or have never heard an organ being played. Listen carefully to the conversation to ensure the discussion is objective and not judgmental. This is not the time to preach one's beliefs but have a broader perspective of various influences on each generation.

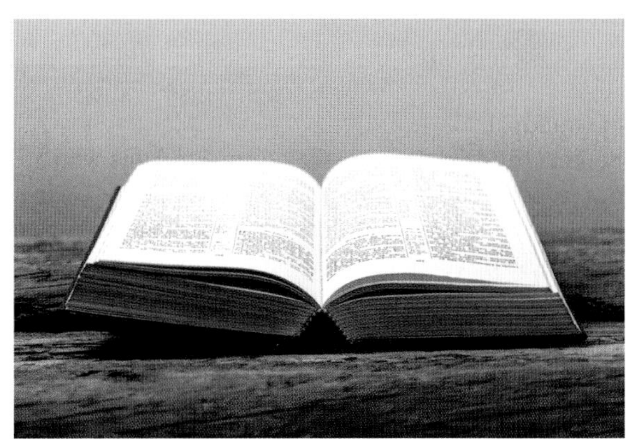

(Oleksandr Bushko/iStock.)

Men and Women

Added to the mix of influences is whether you were/are a man or woman, as each generation saw these roles very differently from what they are today. Women in the military, for example, were treated differently in the

1970s than women in the 1990s, and even those in the 1990s were treated differently from women in today's Armed Forces. While women have had many roles and ranks in their military careers, it has taken time for women to be accepted as part of the military armed forces. Though women can perform many tasks that their male counterparts can, there are other factors the military had to consider, such as being in close quarters with men, the hostile environment men and women would be in during combat, and the political environment. TV shows such as *M*A*S*H* also portrayed women more on the flirtatious side (e.g., "Hot Lips" aka Major Houlihan and the womanizer "Hawkeye" aka Captain Pierce), which contributed to the inuendoes of women being in the military. These shows, while providing humor, also create questions as to whether women should be allowed in the military. However, when reflecting upon the standards, most women were able to bypass the stereotypes and continue to make rank as well as compete with their male counterparts.

Just as the military had to review allowing women in the Armed Forces, religious orders had to relook at female roles and using women to perform tasks that previously were only given to men. Women became priests in some religious faiths and could have their own congregations. While this may sound contemporary and uplifting to some students, others struggle with these new roles, as for them, the woman's place was traditionally in the home and caring for the children. These same students may also struggle with the fact that men can now obtain paternity leave and often stay home and care for the children while their wives (or partners) work. These role reversals can make for good conversations as long as you remain very objective as to the pros and cons of duties and responsibilities. Remember, this is about generational influences, why these roles were assigned to each sex in the first place, and why they have evolved or changed.

Not every culture keeps up with American culture; many retain their own cultural influences, retain their historical perspective, and are not as forgiving with contemporary roles. How women dress, take care of the family, and even their body may be dictated by their culture, religious views, and what the cultural society allows. While some practices may seem barbaric or old-fashioned to Gen Zers, each student should respect other cultures and attempt to maintain an open mind.

Looking at world and current events from the woman's perspective, or a different culture, can be a springboard for a variety of discussions. It can foster empathy and understanding between both men and women, or at least provide a stimulating conversation. Some of your students may be from other cultures and share how they feel about some of the restrictions their culture imposes that are different from American culture (such as arranged marriages, women in politics, and men caring for children). Be sure to keep topics global and steer away from subjects that may be too sensitive, such as war, foreign trade, or immigration. You may tread softly on other subjects such as human trafficking, child slave labor, and subjects where most students can align with one another on similar viewpoints, regardless of their sex.

Sex and Gender

In the current world, these terms often get confused and even mistaken. Sex is used to define the presence of sexual organs at birth; an infant is born either male or female at birth based on these anatomical parts. Gender is the affiliation a person aligns themselves with, such as male, female, or, if they align with the opposite sex, transgender. Gender is often based on an internal awareness and can also be described as gender identity. While this is a brief and noninclusive list or definition, it is enough to realize that terms must correctly be identified so that neither you, nor other students, mistake these terms.

LGBTQ

Many institutions are including lesbian, gay, bisexual, transgender, and questioning (or queer) (LGBTQ) (or some version) in their civility or diversity training. Faculty must be aware of the issues surrounding this population and how to address such issues. While we will not get into what that discussion looks like (as it varies based on each institution), it is important that you are aware of the use of language and reference. One discussion in your class could be very generic, such as "what do these letters mean?" As there is debate about how members of this population refer to themselves (e.g., some prefer to leave off "Q," some consider "Q" as queer, while others consider "Q" as questioning), students may share their perspective or what they have found in their literature review. Members of this population may feel comfortable enough to speak up and share their viewpoint, or you may have an outside speaker come and review this topic. Be cautious that the speaker (or the student) shares the information as *neutral* information, as many students will already have their own opinions based on their culture and belief system. While they try to be open minded, some students may not be as sensitive. The detail of the discussion will be based on what your institution has in place and what it requires. Your job is to simply refer to how our viewpoints of this population stem from our own generation as well as others before us. Even if you are a member of this population or respect that everyone has a choice in their gender and gender affiliation, how you came to this stance has been shaped by generational influences.

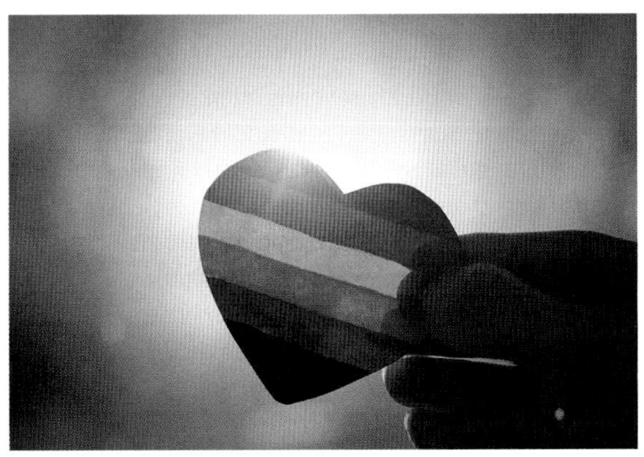

(Roman Didkivskyi/iStock.)

Where Is the Gap?

Though it is probably obvious by now when you have more than one student in a class, you will have varying viewpoints amongst students; however, this gap broadens with the more students you have. More students mean a variety of cultures, different ages, varying generations, and the many variations within each generation. This matrix can become a synthesized collection of unique people who respect one another's perspective. It can also be a hodgepodge of opposing opinions that clash and are difficult to manage. You, as faculty, are the crux of which outcome occurs. Based on how you allow the conversations to be shared, the level of respect or discord present and how far you allow opposing sides to express themselves can make the difference in where the discussion goes. As the facilitator, you must allow diversity and create sensitivity. You must be inclusive but not opinionated. You must be respectful of all but refrain from siding with any. You must remain extremely neutral, which, in urban language, is being Switzerland. The gap that is being referred to is the difference students have in their belief and value structure, their opinions and how they feel. All of these are shaped by the aforementioned attributes and where students do not agree or meet creates a gap.

Ways to Narrow the Gap

Despite your own sensitivity you may find not everyone wants to be Switzerland and will not budge in their beliefs. They simply do not understand how others can behave this way and are appalled that anyone would accept these viewpoints as acceptable. They look to you as the leader, expecting you to raise the flag as referee and deem other opinions unsuitable. As comical as you want to be, now is not the time to throw in the white flag. Provide opportunities for students to journal or present the part of their generation they feel is important (they must present it neutrally). If you feel it is appropriate, have students present the "other" generation and focus on what good this generation has done/is doing for society. Look for things that other generations have contributed which we can now build from—figuratively or literally. From the other perspective, have them share why they get irritated with people outside their generation and why they feel misunderstood. This example of walking in one another's shoes can open their minds to some of the genuine frustrations the other generation has.

Another way to lesson the gap is by combining generations to answer questions such as trivia, music, or events. Games such as *Jeopardy* or some of the other critical thinking exercises shared in Chapter 4 could be useful as people may have different knowledge bases and are able to answer the questions that other generations may not. Be sure to ask questions from their culture, generation, age bracket, or point of reference. Unless you have Centenarians (those who are older than 100 years old) or history buffs in your class, asking questions related to the 1920s may not be appropriate unless it specifically refers to a present-day issue (like measles and immunizations).

Music

A very fun and easy type of game to play regarding generations uses music. Most students enjoy music in some form (especially your musical learners) and can recall popular songs and artists during their generations, and often their parents' or children's generations. The following games can be done in small groups to jumpstart the fun and to show how each generation is needed. However, before you dust off your AC/DC album or get your 8-track player ready to start up again (a scary thought), you may want to review the list of activities. Some of these will open *your* mind to new information; as the leader of the band you must stay unbiased, no matter how much you loathe certain musical genres.

- Compile a list of songs ranging within the generations in your class. Create a playlist of these songs on your smartphone, iPod, or other device. Ask each group to identify the song and the artist, but only play a short piece of the song. Ensure these songs are from a variety of genres (country, rock & roll, jazz, rap) but are mainstream (implying most people from this generation would know this song). Have a few odd ones and offer bonus points if they can guess these less mainstream songs (don't go too far off the mainstream path). Allow points if they guess a similar artist (e.g., *Life Is a Highway* sounds similar whether Tom Cochran or Rascal Flatts sings it, though the latter made it more popular with the movie *Cars*).
- Ask students to pair like-minded artists to form a group based on the name of their band. For example, Queen and Prince, Alabama and the Georgia Satellites, Boston and Chicago, Counting Crows and the Black Crowes … you get the idea. This also can require some critical thinking skills if the relationship between names is not obvious (perhaps Madonna and Judas Priest?).
- Alphabet soup: give students a short time to work together and name one band (along with one song) with each letter of the alphabet. Example: the band A-ha and their song *Analogue*. Depending upon other rules you instill, you may allow them to use the Internet but still complete the task within a brief period of time. Play other music as they are scrambling to get their list, as this can confuse people as they are trying to hear the band in their head.

Caution: if you have members from outside the United States who are not familiar with American music, allow them to be scorekeeper or give them another role, otherwise they may not be able to participate and may feel they are not contributing.

A few simple rules: segregate groups based on their apparent generation to ensure each group has a mix (unless you are having the battle of the generations, assuming you have enough of each generation to make opposing small groups). Songs must be mainstream and have lyrics—no classical music (unless this is a music appreciation class). Songs must be the clean version (unless you pause it before any profanity is sung). Respect is given when listening to the songs, whether it is Tupac, Barry Manilow, Lil' Wayne, or Willie Nelson.

Last rule: don't feel old when students say they love this music because it reminds them of their grandma.

Humor

Throughout the chapters we have focused on introducing humor appropriately during class. If these ideas didn't tickle your funny bone, find something that you think your students would laugh at. When we can laugh at ourselves, we find that we are more alike than different. Perhaps you have an exercise whereby students share what's silly about their generation. Maybe they can more readily identify some of the narrowmindedness, strange opinions, and rigid views that their peers have. Though they may feel bound to defend their generation, it can be refreshing to poke fun at some of the things they do that make you want to be from another generation, or another planet.

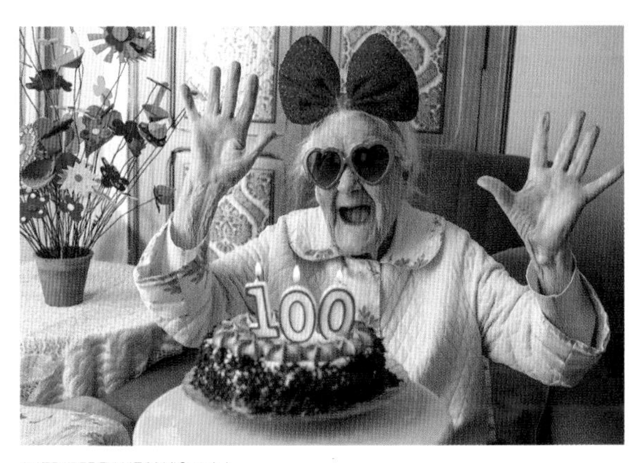

(MEDITERRANEAN/iStock.)

If your institution allows it, have a spirit day whereby students can dress up according to their generation (including cross-dressers). Allow individuality and self-expression but have some rules. All major body parts must be covered, especially breast/chest area, buttocks, midriff/belly area, and students must wear shoes (for safety). Or you can have them dress according to another generation, perhaps one they admire (this is where you may find more vintage clothing from the 1960s, 1920s, or earlier). Allow students to have a potluck from a particular era and enjoy foods that were not completely made from a box or grocery store. Some students may wonder how anyone could survive on a gelatin salad or be surprised that pigs-in-a-blanket and meatballs are still popular 60 years later. This exercise can be especially helpful in a nutrition class, as you dissect the nutritional value of each food, regardless of how gross students think it is.

Another activity is to simply use words or phrases that mean things based on different generations and cultures. Words such as a "45" and "pop" have different connotations as do "tag," "troll," and "poke." These words mean very different things based on generation and culture; have your group find more words and list their various definitions. If they get stumped, you may allow them to Google it—another new term that is both a verb and noun. You can use terms that have been replaced, such as taxis being replaced with Uber and Lyft, and snarky is the new sassy.

Movies and the Media

Like the music games, substitute movies for music and create another fun activity whereby students must recall movies from various generations or the theme of the movie. See how many movies are made with similar themes, like *Tootsie*, *Victor, Victoria*, and *Mrs. Doubtfire*, or *Daddy Day Care*, *Mr. Mom*, and *The Pacifier*. You may also look at movies that were redone with different cast, such as *Steel Magnolias* (made with one all-white cast and redone with an all-black cast), *Barbershop* and *Beauty Shop* (similar movies, though one focuses on male bonding while the other is more female focused). Even if you don't know all the answers (spoiler alert—you never will), your students will, when they work together. Another genre of movies ties in with the LGTBQ population; movies such as *In and Out* and *The Birdcage* were controversial for their time but offered a bit of humor in understanding different gender orientations. Always screen movies before you share them with your class and be sensitive to any student who finds the discussion uncomfortable.

Media is another way to share differences, as older generations grew up with hearing news on the radio, watching TV, or reading the newspaper. Younger generations may have never opened a newspaper, never watched the news on TV, and use Apple TV. Simply starting a conversation for your small groups with: how do you learn about current events? Where do you get your "news" about what's going on in the world today? How do know this information is unbiased and reliable?, can create many hours of discussion. Some students honestly may think that reports from Fox News, CNN, and other media are fact; some students may think they have done their own cross-referencing to ensure the information is legitimate. While there are more neutral media stations and companies/websites that validate information, it is helpful for students to realize this sort of scrutiny takes interest and effort. Just because a parent, friend, spouse, teacher, or social media page says so, doesn't mean it is so.

Show and Tell

This form of learning has not lost its value, as many students are hands-on and visual learners. If you have any old forms of music (vinyl is the new CD) or players (hurrah for hanging on to that 8-track!), bring them in or show a picture of these forms of music/players. You can divide these items into your small groups; ask students to share why this was used, or how it helped the evolution of media. You can even have them use more critical thinking skills and connect the dots: how did the Walkman help create the iPod? What could be the benefits of Apple TV over cable (does anyone have cable TV?)? What were rabbit ears and how do we use that technology now (hint: satellites)? You can also ask why critical thinking skills are important when considering music, media, and movies—are they a sign of the times? A prediction of the future? An opportunity for fantasy or to reveal history? Or something more?

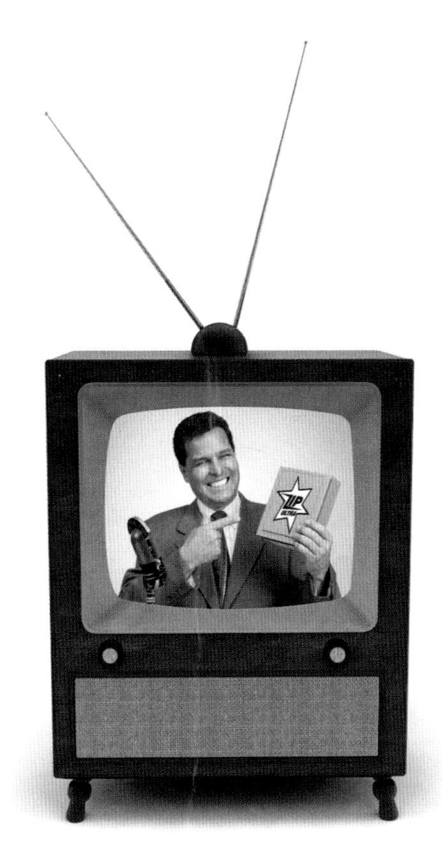

(jgroup/iStock.)

But What Does This Have to Do With Class?

While these activities can help bridge the gap between students, what does it have to do with class? You still must go over the material as outlined in the instructional plan (IP) or syllabus, you still have a certain number of hours that must be covered as well as tests, breaks, review of homework. How does playing songs get you through your "have to teach" list? As we have reviewed in each chapter, student engagement is paramount when considering success. When students use active learning techniques and are engaged, not only are they using more critical thinking skills, they are also increasing their use of Bloom's taxonomy in the areas of applying, evaluating, and creating. Moreover, they are using other skills to work with teammates and must employ other critical thinking and soft skills during such communication. The adage "two brains are better than one" can help offset any negative implication that doing this work is best left for solitary learners; although you can adjust a few exercises to working alone, there is more to the exercise. Working in teams or small groups allows students to get outside of their own understanding of how life is. They can begin to look at varying degrees of acceptance when it comes to different roles, responsibilities, and behavior.

Any class on communication will have to deal with varying perspectives based on generations, gender, culture, and sensitivities. When speaking with clients, patients, or customers, for example, it is important that you understand where they are coming from in order to gain compliance. When students are compassionate about attributes that are not their own, they are better able to work with these clients, patients, and customers and increase both their satisfaction as well as their own confidence. This can close the gap between people and provide trust and a professional relationship—attributes each generation enjoys. Trust is a great foundation that is often lost when dealing with different generations and cultures, unless empathy or compassion is felt. Although these skills seem simple, they may take practice or at least some repetition before they are integrated in one's own behavior. A student who did not grow up with such an open mind or attitude may struggle, although others who were raised in an environment that welcome varying perspectives may have little issue with discussing controversial topics without any bias.

Darth Vader and Mufasa

Remember the exercise whereby students compared and contrasted two fictitious leaders, Darth Vader and Mufasa? We must recognize that—based on each student's personal history and experiences—this discussion could result in spirited debates and varying levels of engagement. Obviously cultural differences, age, world events, and current events will each influence student perceptions. Some students may be unable to compare the kind-hearted, loving Mufasa (*Lion King's* father) to the evil, crazy (former) Jedi who killed people to serve the vile Emperor. A student with an authoritarian, abusive father may be unable to see any positive traits in Darth Vader. Another student without that background who loves movie villains may defend Darth Vader, claiming in the end he chose to put his son's life ahead of universal domination.

They may not see the two leaders as opposites and may struggle with the contrast. To help facilitate the exercise, if you have students who are familiar with the movies and characters and are interested in the activity, you may ask them to role-play the two leaders from different perspectives. Another option for student engagement would be to show clips from the movies that compare and contrast their actions. In a healthcare example, a diabetic patient has lost his father and misses him dearly as his father guided him on his food choices. The dietitian, however, was raised by a single mother and did not have a father figure in his life. The dietitian cannot understand how much the patient relied on his father to maintain compliance with his eating plan; the dietitian sees the patient as non-compliant with his diet, causing his disease to get out of control. Putting yourself in the shoes of the dietitian, how can you empathize with the patient and offer support? What might you would refrain from discussing? Why?

In another example, a young student nurse is working at a community clinic. A 14-year-old patient has come to the clinic complaining of an upset stomach and fatigue. She's accompanied by her grandmother, who has raised her since the mother died 10 years ago. With pride, the grandmother says: "She is a good girl, does well in school, makes friends easily, and works hard." The grandmother has raised the young girl in a household where abstinence before marriage is expected.

The physician orders a urine sample and a few other tests; after conducting an exam, the physician asks that the student nurse stay with the grandmother while the physician speaks to the young girl alone. The physician invites the grandmother back into the exam room, where the granddaughter is crying. The physician reveals that the girl is pregnant. The student nurse must support the physician in educating the girl and her grandmother on pregnancy, options for adoption and/or termination, and sexually transmitted infections (STIs) while remaining objective and not passing judgment.

After your students get a sense of real-life scenarios, they can begin to adjust their thinking and realize that understanding various perspectives will help them, no matter their career path. For example, the young student nurse might better be able to bridge the gap and open the discussion between the grandmother and her granddaughter. Perhaps the student understands how difficult it is for the grandmother to realize that her granddaughter has been having sex. By remaining objective and trying to see the situation through the eyes of two different generations, the student may be able to see both sides. Although the student nurse must remain objective herself, she can still be supportive of the grandmother *and* the patient.

Historical Figures: Fact or Fiction

When reviewing historical figures or famous people, it can stir up a variety of emotions. However, it can also bridge some of the gaps between what you know, what your students know, and what their experiences have been. While some have read of a major event or heard about it from relatives, some lived it or saw firsthand the effects of that event. Gaining various perspectives can be helpful when reviewing how the past has affected our present, and how both can impact our future. While society may want to erase some controversial events or forget abhorrent cruelties done to people (based on their perspective), we must learn from these situations. While indeed there have been horrible events in the world, what traits have been the same? This can be an excellent way to get various generations, cultures, and your mix of students to discuss common traits, both negative and positive, that people have—regardless of their generation or current status of society. Which ones are ones that we want more of nowadays? Which ones are ones that we want to perpetuate (e.g., compassion, kindness, etc.)? What do those traits look like? Are there some human traits that have not changed? We can decrease the gap in our generations when we decrease our disdain for differences and increase our respect for such differences. Tolerance is the ability to raise one's ability to "endure" something without having a consequence. While many people consider tolerance a negative word, it is neutral. If we tolerate kindness, we increase our vulnerability. If we tolerate love, we crave more—in fact. We may never get enough love.

Just as there is tolerance for abuse, drugs, and negative connotations, there can also be tolerance for positive things. This can open another discussion, based on the material you are presenting. By valuing each member of society, now and those before us, we respect individuality; not just for the Mufasas of the world, but also for the Darth Vaders. That does not mean we agree with Vader's tactics, but if we are to be a loving people, we love all. We don't pick and choose. Can we, as a society, community, or world, love (or tolerate) *everyone*?

In addition to our historic figures we also have other iconic figures. Out of a necessity to believe in something bigger, Superman, Wonder Woman, and Batman were created. Many of your Baby Boomers will recall reading the first comics of both Marvel and DC, as well as many other superheroes that were turned into movies. Gen Xers will appreciate other heroes such as the *Six Million Dollar Man* and the *Bionic Woman*, as well the evolution of science fiction (*Star Trek* and *Star Wars*). These shows, movies, and comics have gone to another level of interest with conventions and role playing of various figures. This allows various generations to discuss movies, characters, or eras of different iconic figures, even from a philosophical nature. From the Socratic method, ask students why did we need these? What have these figures done for society? For men? For women? For children? What has the government done to support these figures in society?

One of the most engaging activities to bridge the gap is to have students discover answers to very vague questions. By using the Socratic method and probing, students must continuously use critical thinking skills. Indeed, there are no right answers, but everyone's opinion. Many exercises have been shared as to how to initiate conversations that span across the generations. Even simple definitions of what constitutes "men's work" versus "women's work" now and with prior generations can stir up a great deal of chatter. Again, there are no right answers, but varying perspectives based on gender, culture, and generations.

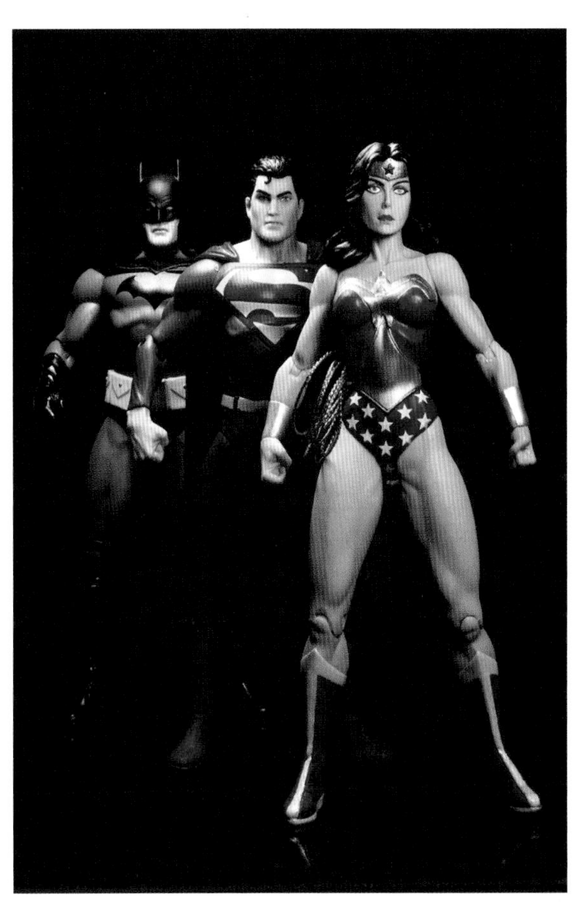

(BrendanHunter/iStock.)

Journal: Self-reflection

1 Which generation do you identify most with?

____

2 What other generations have you lived with?

____

____

3. How do you feel about generations outside your own—share your perspective of the Silent Generation, Baby Boomers, Gen Xers, Millennials, and Gen Zers:

4. What culture do you most associate with?

5. What other cultures have you lived with?

6. Considering other cultures, list at least four cultures (outside your own) and your view of that culture. What do you see as their strengths? What do you see as a valuable trait from this culture? How did you come to this belief?

7. What were some primary events (social, community, or worldly) that occurred during your childhood or that you recall?

8. What experience or any training have you had with:
   a. Veterans/military:

b. LGBTQ:

9 What are your own personal spiritual or religious beliefs? What exposure have you had with other beliefs?

10 How do you view the roles of men and women? What are your views of transgender people?

11 Several games and activities have been shared to reduce the gap between students. The following exercises are suggestions that can help facilitate this goal. The questions below will help you brainstorm on these ideas; you will have a chance to come up with your own ideas later in this journal.

a. Music: which exercise resonated with you from the ones listed? How would you roll this out with your class? What songs or activities would you include?

b. Humor is a great way to bridge different generations. What exercises, activities, or games would you include in your class? List three different games or activities (you may include the ideas suggested).

c. Movies span generational ties; many have been re-created from earlier generations. List three activities you may use to incorporate movies and the media and how both have shaped our society.

d. Show and tell can get crazy when older generations bring in items for which their younger peers have no reference point. Think of a few items that you would want or may have yourself that you could use (if not the item, a picture of the item). What discussion could surround these items? What reference point would these items have with your class topic?

e. Historical figures have shaped our version of reality—both fictional and real ones. List five figures that you would want to refer to and their influence on our society.

f. If you had the chance to invite any six people (alive or dead, real or fictional) to be a guest speaker in your class—who would they be? What would you want them to discuss or share?

g. What were the roles of men and women in your household growing up? How have they changed in your current household? What conversations could your students have that would relate their own upbringing and viewpoint of these roles to the subject matter you are teaching. Use your own critical thinking skills to come up with at least four activities whereby the roles of men and women currently impact our society based on your course topics.

h. As mentioned, tolerance can be used in a positive way. In your opinion, what should our students be tolerant of in order to form a better "planet"?

i. Civility has been referred to as a lost art, or at least one that is waning. Do you agree with this statement? What are some activities you can use to help promote civility in your class?

12 Now is your time to come up with a unique game that can bridge the gap between generations. Try to be as specific as possible so that you will have the details mapped out when it is time to roll it out!

Each age, it is found, must write its own books; or rather,
each generation for the next succeeding.
Ralph Waldo Emerson

Chapter 9

Self-assessment and Improvement

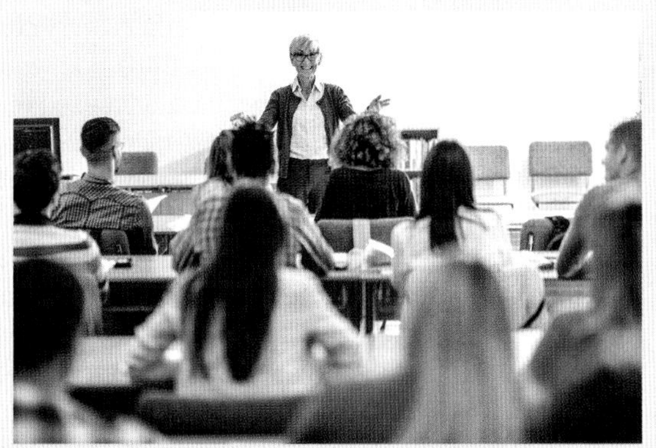

(skynesher/iStock.)

While the previous eight chapters have been designed to prepare you for the classroom, this chapter will cause you to stop and reflect on how well you have done in the classroom. This chapter should be reviewed after teaching a few classes, or at least one course. Having taught a class or two, there are things that you can begin to evaluate within your style, your approach, and most of all, your effectiveness. Let's start back at the beginning—you wanted to be a teacher. Do you still feel that way? Hopefully you do, but you may feel that you need a tune up, which is what this chapter is all about. No one is perfect out of the chute, and no one remains great without a bit of reevaluation. All teachers need to perform ongoing self-assessments in order to maintain a fresh perspective, be effective, and be realistic.

As you were teaching, did you find there were days you wondered if you had planned a course at all? Did you feel frustrated, overwhelmed, or lost? Perhaps you felt that teaching was not what you thought it was. Did some things go right, and others go wrong? Welcome to the field of teaching. Despite the hours you have spent planning, preparing, reviewing, and reviewing again, there are days when nothing you planned will go well, and other days when you wonder if you should be teaching at all. These are very normal reactions to the profession, they can happen in each setting, and can make any teacher feel like throwing in the towel. The truth is, those who choose not to throw in the towel will survive, get better, and guide others. Teaching requires a great deal of humility, as what you thought was well crafted and put together may or may not work and you may have to start over. You may lose momentum, get sidetracked, or even steer off course. As mentioned in previous chapters, this is to be expected. Even though you are human, you are also working with a variety of other people (peers, managers, an institutional board, regulatory bodies, and your institution's plethora of folks), plus students. Each of these people have different requirements which are not necessarily in alignment with your plans, nor do they meet your expectations. While, in fact, you must meet their expectations (even if they may not be in total alignment) you must also be in sync with yourself.

Despite a little bit of humility, it is important to remain objective about your teaching. Just as we reviewed best practices for your course, we must evaluate whether you are using best practices and evaluate your methodology. While there will be more self-reflection at the end of this chapter, we will review some basic points to ensure you are applying these principles. We will review all aspects from the start to the end, review previous chapters, and determine the areas where you can improve. Before we do, let's consider your feelings. In the first chapter you were asked when you got the gumption or inspiration to be a teacher. Along with that spark also came a preconceived notion of what teaching should be like. Perhaps you expected that you would always know what to say, or that your years in the industry would help guide you. If you are well versed in your field and have conducted many training sessions, you may have expected students to be more interested in listening to you or hearing your stories as they relate to their field. You may have felt that students have a requirement to behave in class, take notes, and have an earnest desire to learn, as they are in a diploma or degree program. Perhaps you are surprised at the way students behave or the cavalier attitude they seem to possess, despite the fact that they (or someone) are spending a great deal of money for their education. You may be disheartened when you approach your peers or manager to learn that your students are no more special, unique, or smarter than other classes. Perhaps you feel the sense of failure as you were not able to meet the mark or give 100%. If any of these rings a slight bell, welcome (again) to the field of teaching.

In reviewing your class, what was the end of the class day like? Did students want to leave early, were they bored? How did you feel? Were there several areas you felt you did not get a chance to review? Were you done with what you planned in half the class time? Did you even get to do what you planned? If you got off course, what happened? Did you go off on a tangent on other information? Did students lure you away from your main talking points? Did they have a different agenda than yours? Perhaps you felt that you were in a crucible of nonstop questioning or even arguments; maybe you thought you were starring in your own version of the *Call of the Wild*? There are many things that can introject themselves in a day, based on you, on your students, and on life. Even the most prepared and seasoned faculty can have days that end up totally different from what they planned and how they started the day. Don't get too discouraged but do step back and review what happened. To do that, we will go backward to determine common areas of derailment.

Audience

When considering your audience, did you have a chance to meet with them prior to the first day of class? What was your impression when you did meet them? What preset judgments did or do you have? Before you claim you have no judgments, biases, or preconceived notions, if you found yourself disappointed at all, you had *some* expectations. If you did not have *any* expectations, you would not be disappointed. What were your expectations? Think about that for a moment—you wanted your class to ... you looked forward to your students ... whatever you fill in these blanks with, realize that indeed you have unmet expectations. Are these expectations realistic? Whether you expected your students to behave a certain way or you expected yourself to do a better job, it is based on an internal desire. Do you have a desire to please others (very common in teaching)? Perhaps you didn't think you would stumble or thought you could be more organized once you got into the class. How did the students respond?

Content should be related to the audience, and it often takes a few days to realize what they know and what they don't know. Were you prepared with this analysis—did you know their familiarity with the subject? Were you able to ascertain this familiarity quickly, or did you struggle? Even if your first few days of teaching went well, this ongoing question runs deep in each class, as you will constantly be gauging what your students know. Once you understand their knowledge base you can direct your teaching more effectively. Without this knowledge and the ability to plan accordingly, it may feel like shooting a target while blindfolded. You keep hoping that you will hit the bull's-eye, but eventually you simply just want to hit any spot on the target. This is not only frustrating, but also ineffective. Best practices do encourage and allow minor adjustments along the way, but prior planning can prevent needing so many adjustments. It cannot be stressed enough how important it is that you know your audience. Knowing your audience does not mean you have social hour each day getting to know your students' personal lives, where they live, or how many kids they have. It does mean that you observe their behavior, you ask what educational- and work-related experience they have had. It often entails taking some notes, not to point out specifics of any one student, but to see overall what mix you have. Though you can do a lot of activities whereby students are the leaders of their learning, this reconnaissance requires you be at the helm. You need to direct this inquiry, though you can be creative in how you acquire the information. Remember, you are not looking for individual nuances, but general trends with your students; as an audience, where do you need to guide them?

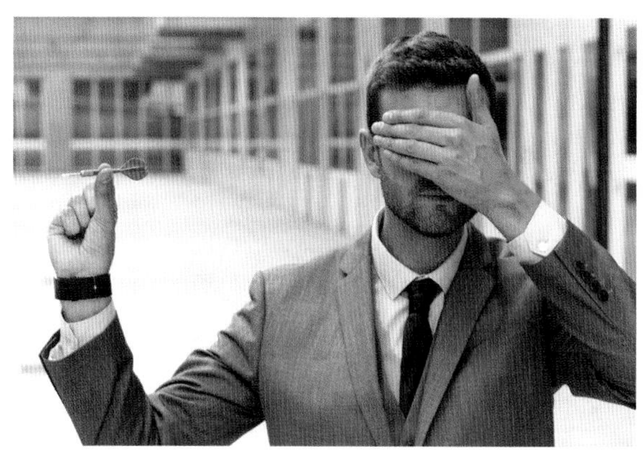
(ajr_images/iStock.)

Who's Managing Whom?

In previous chapters we went over important factors regarding diversity, inclusion, and ensuring students were engaged and involved. Did all students participate? Were there students who tried to take over, or others who did not participate at all? Did some leave class and never return, or pretend to step out for a bathroom run or phone call? Did you feel that the monkeys were running the zoo? It can be a bit unsettling to have to monitor and attempt to control a classroom environment (although we all know we can control only ourselves). You may have one or two strong-willed students who take charge of the classroom discussions and continuously speak out; stating they are speaking for all. These students often feel the need to share their viewpoint as it is their right to freedom of speech; often this "sharing" is at the cost of other students, as they may not feel the same way. Always respect each student but remind the more vocal ones that you'd like to hear from other students. This may even take a few reminders, especially if other students remain quiet. Again, even silence can be loud. To foster respect, let students know that everyone has the right to share but not everyone may want to; if there is quiet time, we will respect that, too.

In considering the demographics of your students, what mix do you have? A variety of ages, generations, cultures, and genders? Perhaps you can divide and conquer; allow some small groups to fit together based on two commonalities; allow them to share collectively. Did you rotate the members of the group to ensure each person has a role such as scribe, researcher, or presenter? Did you have the presenter use a whiteboard (or a wall pad) and have one person write the summary for all to see? Did you feel that you used all resources in these classes? In this scenario, you can ask questions to get to know students' backgrounds more fully and base it on some common themes. This can help you plan better, as you may discover perspectives you weren't previously aware of. As an example, let's say you are trying to learn a bit more about a class you are teaching to a group of Medical Assisting (MA) students. Most of them are younger (in their 20s) and all are female. There is a mix of cultures and ethnicities, so you ask them to divide up into groups of similar ethnic backgrounds. To keep it fun they can make a group name if desired. There are four groups, who name themselves: the Oreos (mix of black and white students), the Zan Wok (Asian students; "Zan" means supportive), Ananda (Indian students; "Ananda" means happy), and the Sexy Enchiladas (Hispanic students). Immediately you see that two groups went for funny names, while the other two went for names based on their culture. Using the Socratic method, you begin asking several questions to determine their approach to education. You discover that the blacks, whites, and Hispanics have had a similar class before, and have worked as a certified nursing assistant (CNA). They see this class as a fun opportunity to learn more but also feel it's a breeze; they expect to get an "A." Many students in these three groups are young, and about half of them are single moms. On the flipside, the Zan and Ananda groups are providing for their larger families. Many have never been employed in health care but have been caregivers for dying grandparents. The Zan group is quieter and tries to take copious notes, having had no prior background. The Ananda group is very social but doesn't quite fit in with the other groups. They have strong family ties and can identify with the Asian group. However, the concept of being a single mother is strange. The Ananda group is studious and wants to learn more, but also feel if it doesn't work out, they can switch to a different program. The other groups fear that they could not provide for their family if they fail this course.

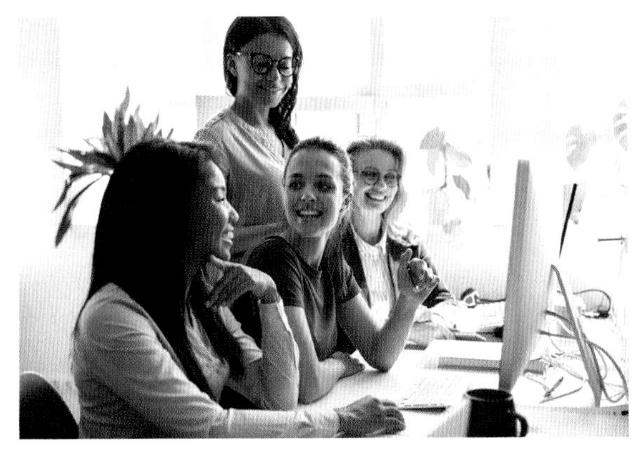

(fizkes/iStock.)

Just from this exercise, you have learned who values their education and why. The three groups (other than Ananda) need this class (from their perspective). Their motivation may be based on fear, and their drive is to care for others. The Ananda group has a different focus and may even seem selfish or standoffish, even though they are social. This gives you more information when deciding what activities to do, where to put your focus, and how to bring out the talents of each group. There may be times you wish to maintain these groups in their separateness, and other times you mix it up. How do the single moms feel when there is a lot of homework assigned? Did they even do the homework? Did the Asian students understand it? Do they each have a place to do their work at home? What interruptions are going on at home? These more neutral discussions can allow students from different backgrounds to meld, as they have commonalities. However, it also gives you feedback as you have learned quickly what other struggles they have. Perhaps you need to refocus your day and allow some time to review homework before the end of class; maybe help students who have other chores or children to prioritize. You can use peer mentoring if students are open, or even as a class discussion. A nonthreatening exercise (using yourself) can illustrate prioritization—even in a comical way.

Let's say you use the example of coming home to a house where your three children are. You have hurried home and didn't stop to use the restroom; you want to make a beeline for the bathroom but notice a strange smell. You swing by the kitchen and notice a pot of pasta is boiling over all over the stove; you hear your infant crying in his room (you think he's in the crib). You call out for your teenage son who was watching his siblings and hear nothing. Your middle daughter comes running in with the dog, covered in mud, and continues to run through the house screeching. At that exact moment your cell phone goes off and it is your son's friend. What do you do first? Why? Different groups may have different ideas or rationales, as there is no correct answer. However, some reasons are better than others. The muddy dog, though exasperating to clean up, is not the priority. Your infant (unless he is safe in his crib) and the stove are safety issues. Of course, you have got to run to the bathroom, but whether or not you choose to is another discussion (some students will defer to doing laundry if you have an accident). And your son? Finding him may not be the first thing you do but it is a priority, as this is unusual behavior for him. The fact that his friend calls causes you concern—is he with the friend? And why is the friend calling *you*—is there an accident or emergency?

Doing these types of exercises allows you to also see what is important to your students; what is important to your students can further guide you and help you meet your mark when teaching. Perhaps the first few minutes of class they are more concerned with checking in on the family and are late. You ask that we start class on time (be here by 0800) but the first 10 minutes will be on decompressing. It allows students to call and check in, come back to the reality that they are in class, and center themselves for you. If you had expected to walk into class and find them ready to start but then took another 30 minutes trying to get everyone focused, you will need to relook at what is causing them to be distracted. Until you can gain everyone's full attention and willingness to participate, you can be the most exciting and engaging teacher and you will not gain any momentum. Consider the example when you came home to so many (potential) disasters; if a friend stopped by and wanted to take you out to dinner, you couldn't even focus on what she was asking until all the other emergencies were "handled," or at least you realized what was going on. Once everything was calmed down and taken care of, and all children accounted for, you may need a dinner out—but not in the middle of the crisis.

Planning

We reviewed the many things you had to plan for prior to your class; however, there are some things you simply cannot plan for. Just as in this example, you thought you had everything planned out—your son was to watch the children for 3 hours until you got home (he does this every Friday). He had to make macaroni and cheese (something he has done with your supervision and done well), along with raw carrots and leftover chicken. He is very responsible and often cares for his younger siblings. Your infant is a very happy child and rarely cries, except when he is hurt or if there is a stranger around. However, both your eldest son and your daughter know how to be safe with and around the baby, and ensure he is tended to while sleeping and when he is awake. Your daughter loves to explore outdoors and usually follows the rule of no running in the house (let alone running with a muddy dog). And how did they get muddy? It's a clear, warm day. In addition to planning a simple afternoon, you also alerted the neighbor Mrs. Wesley that you would be home a bit later today and could she just check in to make sure everything was alright? Your cell phone number was plastered on the kitchen wall, bedroom and bathrooms, and with every neighbor. How could it be that everything you planned for went up in smoke?

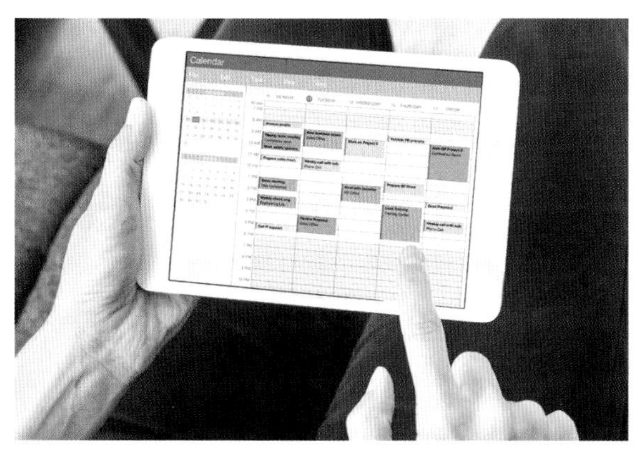

(NicoElNino/iStock.)

Planning decreases poor performance, but no amount of planning can cover every "what if." That is why ongoing evaluation of yourself, your expectations, and your interpretations should be reviewed. Maybe you forgot that your son started football practice this Friday at 5 p.m. (you arrived at 5:10 p.m.). Perhaps the friend was calling to remind you that your son was with him (as he left his phone at home). Mrs. Wesley thought she'd help in between and wanted to start dinner for the younger ones, but she had to check on the crying infant—who had a very dirty diaper. She doesn't hear very well and didn't realize the infant had been crying before she walked in. Your daughter was trying to give the dog a bath and the hose slipped out of her little hands. No one did anything wrong, and indeed everyone was trying to do as they were told, as per your plans. Life is full of "oops" and things we didn't plan for. Teaching doesn't excuse the "oops" in life; in fact, it seems at times to perpetuate them. Don't be too hard on yourself when things don't go according to plan. Do, however, keep your eye on the goals and objectives.

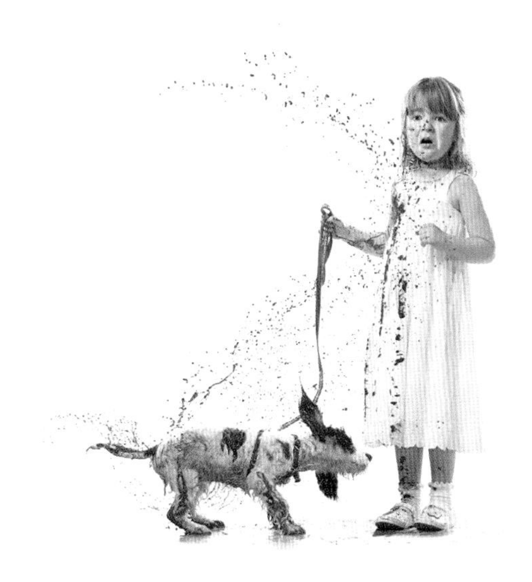

(sturti/iStock.)

Did You Remember the Goals?

Despite the "oops," were the goals achieved or are they still achievable? If your son indeed is at football practice, your infant is fine (now that he has a very clean diaper, despite the fact he has no clue who the lady is who changed him), and your daughter and dog can both get a bath (outside), you can be thankful all is well. A bit messy perhaps, but nothing that can't be cleaned up later. In fact, you call your friend and ask that you order take out and she bring it over, while you both visit and let the children enjoy themselves. The goal: you worked late while your children were cared for. What about the objectives? Safe children were the priority; having fed and clean children are the second priorities (being fed having slightly more importance than being clean). Happy children are desirable but not required. Considering these goals and objectives, they were all met. A few adjustments were made, as your son's job to take care of his younger siblings was overshadowed by his need to be at football practice. On the flip side, you want to ensure he can make decisions and maintain his responsibilities. In this case (and in his mind) he did by making it to practice, calling his friend to alert you, and asking Mrs. Wesley to cover for him.

The same is true for your class. At the end of the day or the week, while it did not go as planned, did you meet the goals and objectives? Go back to the lesson plan (LP) and instructional plan (IP). What did you have to teach? What did you want to teach? What was negotiable (in retrospect)? If you could plan again for this class, what would you include? What would you change? Ongoing evaluation is crucial to ensure that you keep your eyes on the goal and objectives. Even when you get off track, are pulled in other directions, or want to scratch your LP and start over, you must get back to the simplest point: what outcomes are you looking for? What did you achieve? What did you miss? What can you do to meet these missed areas (chances are there are a few minor changes, but a total overhaul is not needed)? Does it simply require a different perspective (on your behalf) or do you need some help?

Student Engagement and Critical Thinking

When considering your class, maybe it went very well, and everyone had fun. They thoroughly enjoyed your teaching style and can't wait for the next class. However, you notice that after the first test, everyone failed. What went wrong? Student engagement, though important for active learning, is not just about engagement. Making sure the activities are engaging but also focused on the material and meeting objectives are just as important. Over the previous eight chapters, several exercises have been shared and encouraged; hopefully they can jump start your own creativity. However, they also need to be appropriate. Some classes do not encourage certain activities or any activity. If you must review an in-depth topic in a very short amount of time, there may be no room for games. If you have a guest speaker and a pop quiz, along with a mini lecture, again, there may not be enough room in the day for *Jeopardy*. Deciding what activities to use and when to use them is important—did you plan too much? Did your activities have more to do with teambuilding than learning the material? Did the material you covered miss the material that was required in the objectives?

You also must consider your time. Did you give yourself enough time to plan these appropriate activities? While you must meet objectives, you also need to allow the time it takes to create the adjoining activities. Sometimes, after planning the activity, you may realize it doesn't fit with the lecture presentation and could possibly be saved for later. Suppose you created a few games on the material you are presenting on HIV (the human immunodeficiency virus). As you reflect on this subject, you realize that this subject stirs up many emotions, as it cross-references other subjects which deal with gender, sex, death, religious beliefs, and culture. Your game is more appropriate perhaps for a general discussion of sexually transmitted infections (STIs) or non–sexual-related diseases. This can be a relief when it comes time to present STIs, but you will have to relook at your topic on HIV and determine other more appropriate activities that can allow students to share emotions on the related subjects. Also, you may not have read up on current practices, drugs, and treatment, and may need more prep time on statistics and what the Centers for Disease Control and Prevention (CDC) says. This is a good time to engage students in discovering related topics, but you need to have some answers to ensure you are directing them correctly. Indeed, the CDC has myriad related information, data, and statistics, but navigating through their website can take hours—a fact you would already know if you had a chance to preview the website. Having done your homework, however, you could tell students to look in a specific area on the site and drill down to the information you want them to find.

This is where your own critical thinking comes into play as you discern where they can find valuable and pertinent information, instead of wasting time digging through unrelated material.

Student engagement can often take on different perspectives based on your subject material. While faculty often enjoy the game and fun activities, they may be doing it to gain support of their students. As mentioned, student engagement is not about gaining popularity or competing with Mrs. Cleaver, Teacher of the Year. The tidiness of your classroom and smiles on your students faces isn't why you went into teaching; if it is, you need to reconsider your goals. Visualize students on a pathway, you are the coach, guiding them. Learning requires that you direct students to where the goal is, not by holding their hand but by telling them, showing them, and inspiring them—they must do the walking, and whatever other work is required. How did you guide your class? Did you mentor and inspire; or perhaps you coached them to reach a goal or objective. Did you take them step by step through each phase in the process? Sometimes too much direction interrupts a student's engagement, as it diminishes the need for discovery. Students want to be involved but don't need to be shown everything. Much like that buffet in Chapter 4—you want to entice them and allow them to eat so that they are satiated, but never satisfied. Always persuade them in their quest for more but never give them all the answers. Remember, this is what makes people lifelong learners, including yourself. We will review this more in Chapter 10 but just realize that you are never "done" with learning.

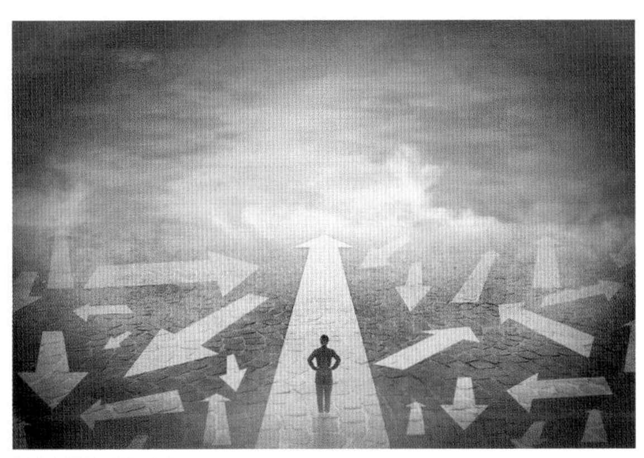

(Bulat Silvia/iStock.)

While you may have been off on student's engagement, did you instill a few critical thinking exercises? Did you stimulate their minds and ask questions that provoked new pursuits, or did you just show them the answers? Did you leave them hungry or did you end their meal? Perhaps you got stumped on critical thinking activities and fell short of ones that were stimulating. Maybe you don't understand how to use critical thinking in the class based on your subject material. These areas are good to reflect on and share with your mentor. Don't be too hard on yourself; if you are not used to critical thinking exercises it can be difficult at first. However, once you start seeing things through that lens you will realize there many examples of how to use critical thinking, in any class, on any subject. Life is full of idiosyncrasies, things that simply don't make sense. Why are we redundant with our words, like an ATM machine (ATM = automatic teller *machine*), past history (is there a future history?), 12 midnight or 12 noon (why even use "12?"; it is either midnight or noon)? There are other areas that simply don't make sense—like Braille on a drive-up ATM; even though it is a requirement of the Americans With Disabilities Act (ADA) and federal regulations, one would question how a blind person would drive up to an ATM. These bits of trivia and thought-provoking questions use critical thinking and can rouse many students to continue to ask more questions. Once they are asking questions, (and you are answering with more questions), you are using the Socratic method to promote critical thinking. Congratulations!

Assessments

Ongoing check-ins are imperative; there is no better way than a periodic question asking, "does this make sense?" Whether at the end of the day or a pause during a lecture, checking in with your students allows you to redirect quickly. However, it may not be as effective if students say they are understanding, able to follow along, and don't have any more questions. What will make the difference is when you conduct actual assessments. Whether it is a pop quiz, or an actual test, these assessments are needed for you to make the necessary adjustments. You need to decide how many assessments are needed to qualify that you are on track.

To Quiz or Not to Quiz?

As mentioned in Chapter 7, assessments give us the gauge to determine whether we, as faculty, are on target. There are many assessments but introducing them at optimum opportunities is crucial; these are check points to redirect faculty and give pertinent feedback to students. So, did you have enough quizzes? Do you have feedback on how students are doing? Is there empirical evidence as to how they comprehend the material? What other measures do you have to assess their understanding? Can you do a quick survey or some pop quizzes? A demonstration or presentation? How do *you* know your students understand the lecture you've given, or the activities you have presented? If you had to vouch for them, could you? Based on what fact? These factors can help you as you navigate whether or not you are on course. *If* you feel that students can capture the appropriate information and your assessments reveal that they are on par, then continue on track. However, if students are struggling, redirect yourself and try something different. Check it out—did that make more sense? If not, try something even more different—did that help? Is it muddier or more clear? What else can the students benefit from? What other resources can you pull in from the Internet or your peers to help? While students feel that quizzes and tests are the be all and end all of their fate within education, the reality is that many other aspects of assessments can give faculty better feedback; we simply need to think outside the box ourselves and be creative. Ask yourself whether you should add another quiz, revise your current quiz, or don't do quizzes at all. You will find the perfect point in which to add (or delete) quizzes once you get a rhythm to your own best practices. However, such finesse takes time. As you are consistently looking at your students to ensure they are hitting the target, you are also being looked at by your students to determine if you are their advocate.

Best Practices and the Gap

In his song, *Turn the Page*, Bob Seger refers to life on the stage. This is a song about someone who is constantly being looked at to see whether they measure up; it also refers to what life is like on the road (for perhaps a band, an acting troupe, or even a teacher). He speaks of constantly being watched, scrutinized, and evaluated. He refers to the fatigue, the sheer exhaustion, the constant feeling that you are under a microscope. Quietly you accept the fact that you are on the road, up on the stage, and playing the star again. In his song Seger speaks of being in the spotlight, and how much you surrender as you give to others. Teaching is much like being on stage; you are constantly "on." Your audience (students) is always watching, perpetually determining if you passed muster. Whether this is a reality or simply what you feel, it can be very real, as you are always on stage—ready to "perform." Even Shakespeare said "all the world is a stage"; we are always subject to the perception of others. Do you feel that you are constantly being evaluated? *Do* you pass muster? In whose eyes? Who decides what has worked and what doesn't? How do you know if it worked?

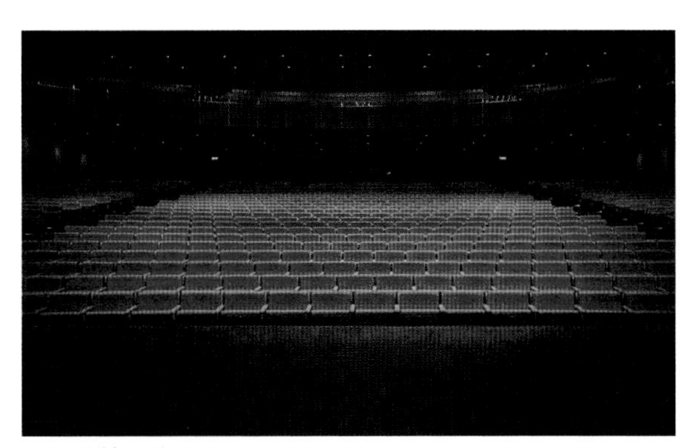

(101cats/iStock.)

Going back to assessments, and whether or not you met the mark, think about what really counts. Remember that the IP is the golden rule; was that, at least, met? What else was met—perhaps some casual goals or informal expectations? How did your summative assessments go? Along the way what did students tell you? What was the result of your student surveys? If it all reflected on your teaching style, perhaps you may need to relook at a few areas. However, if students are not passing, why is that so? What is preventing them from reaching that goal? How effective were you in your instruction? Did you actually focus on the IP goal, or another goal you had in mind?

Best practices imply that you use what has been known as effective in the teaching industry and repeat it to the best of your ability and the best outcome for your students. Students at one institution may not score their professor the same as the professor in a different institution, based on what the goal is. Your goal and that of your students absolutely must be in alignment, based on what the institutional goals are for that course. Outcomes and benchmarks are often reported to regulatory agencies, and if you teach at a different level than prescribed, or on a whim, you might jeopardize your institution's standing. Obviously, this risk is not worth it for a personal sense of academic freedom. It is always best to use best practices; measurable quantities that fall in alignment with your IP. Considering these established guidelines, you can defer to outside practices that support what you're trying to teach. Using prescribed curriculum also supports you when a student wants to argue that the class isn't fair or questions why they must learn certain aspects; the objectives as designed and approved by the institution and regulatory bodies provide the perfect (and correct) answer. This fact can deflate any negative energy that may be directed at you for making the class or tests in a way that doesn't meet students' expectations. Maybe those Oreo and Sexy Enchilada students are upset to find the course was not as easy as they thought, and they may not earn an "easy A."

Where's That Gap?

So where is the gap? Is it between your expectations and that of your institution? Do you feel disconnected? Or do you think you are way out of touch? Perhaps you have a great deal of information on the subject but fall short of how to deliver it? Or maybe you did a good job, but not great. Regardless of how wide or small that gap is, chances are that a gap exists. This is not the time to act like an ostrich; even if you feel depressed you need to get your head out of the sand and realize you must address this gap. If you don't focus on the obstacles that are creating that gap, the gap will increase. Whether it is a gap in generations between you and your students, a gap between your expectations and your students' and/or your institution's, or a gap in how you perform, you must acknowledge the gap. After it is acknowledged, you must address how the gap came into being and what you will do to shorten that gap. The more you can do this, the better you will feel that you are connecting with your students; moreover, the better your students will reach the desired outcomes. While it may take some creative, albeit critical thinking on your part, it is well worth the effort.

What Resources Did You Need?

One thing to always consider is the resources you need to be a great, effective teacher. You are not going to do it without plugging into a few resources, adding some tools to your toolbox, or looking outside (or inside, as Socrates would say) yourself. You must understand that teaching does not come with an all-inclusive manual—even this handbook, despite its many ideas, does not contain every idea you can or should have. Students change, education evolves, institutions vary, and you must be on the cutting edge—looking for the next opportunity to keep up with the changes. So, what else do you need? Perhaps you need to learn more and need to observe a teacher with best practices? Or attend a conference or a webinar? Have you spent enough time reviewing the material, the book, or the IP? Did you put enough time into *understanding* the objectives, even though you are aware of what they are? Do you need more ideas on how to consolidate the material? Maybe you needed more direction?

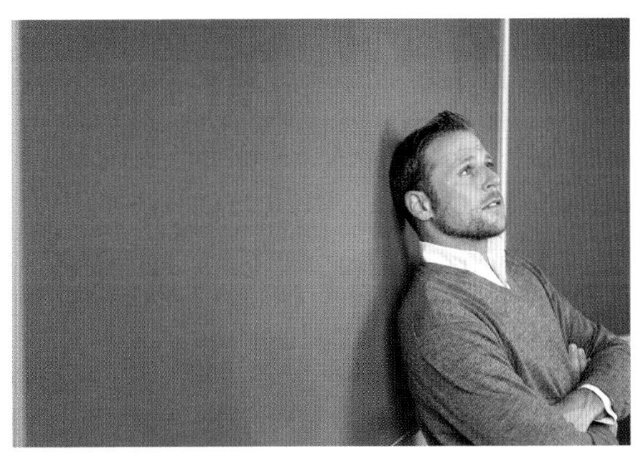

(stockfour/iStock.)

Often faculty feel they need more time. They wonder if they can be adequately prepared with only a few days or weeks to prepare. They need to work more on the PowerPoint (PPT) presentation or handouts and ensure they have covered the material. These factors, which are important, are not always the priority. As mentioned, PPT is the least preferred method of instruction to ensure active learning is taking place; handouts, though helpful, can be done months ahead of time and should be used in conjunction with the activity. If you have reviewed the objectives, the tests, and have the right tools you should be able to clearly identify what else is needed to meet your mark. Somehow, you got lost. What happened? What do you think (other than time) you needed in order to be better prepared? Perhaps better time management? Perhaps a practice round? Think about that further as you look back; as the adage goes, "hindsight is 20/20." When looking back you may start seeing trends in your own gaps.

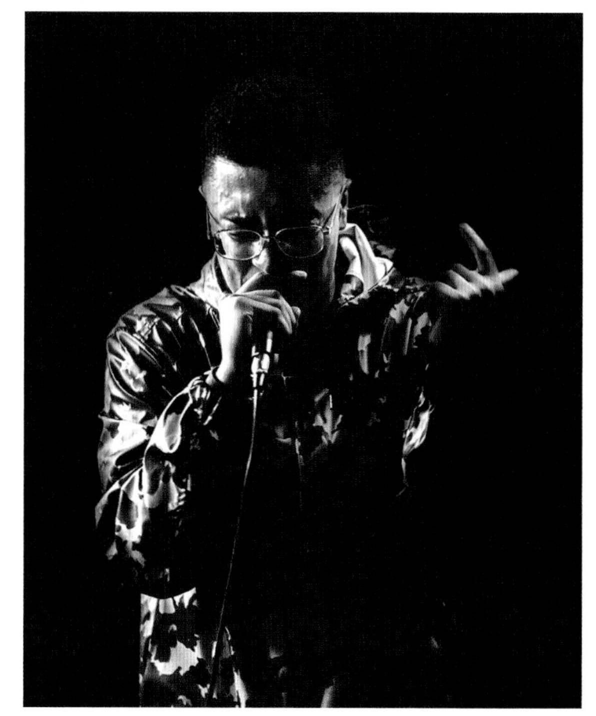

(vyasphoto/iStock.)

What Went Wrong?

When you consider each activity, you may begin to see shortcomings and have a greater awareness of your teaching. For example, you may have tried music but realized the vast difference in your kind of music and that of your students. Are you stuck with Martha and the Vandellas? Did you think everyone would enjoy listening to your AC/DC tapes; maybe you felt that switching to Mötley Crüe was the (wrong) answer? Were you offended by artists such as Tupac or Lil' Wayne? Maybe you did not find any enjoyment with games, let alone having to create them. It is not unusual, based on the differences between you and your students, that there may be some discrepancies in what version of games may be considered fun or appropriate. Even if you don't prefer playing or creating games, did you get a sense your students liked the fact that you attempted it? Maybe you didn't score on *Family Feud*, but they were able to learn a great deal. Can you accept the fact that students learn in ways different from you? Have you begun to realize that your ways may need freshening up?

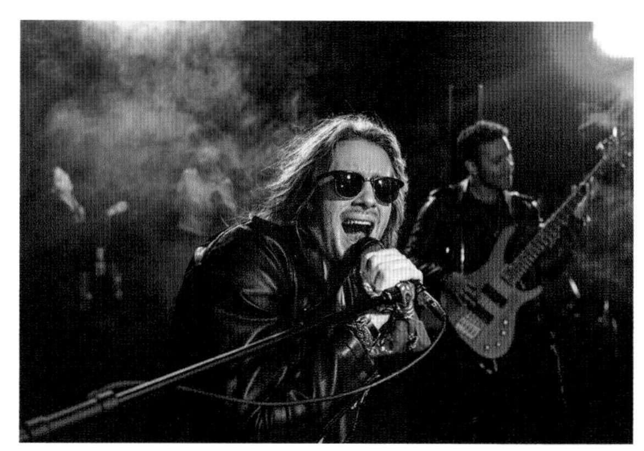

(LightFieldStudios/iStock.)

Perhaps you eagerly embrace games and love the idea of using technology. You appreciate the fact that some students are savvier and into the higher tech industry. You and most of your students connect on a new wave and you are energized by their enthusiasm—but you received a complaint that a student feels overwhelmed and accuses you of playing favorites. You are curious how anyone could see this, as you try your best to maintain a neutral playing field. The fact of the matter is simple: if even one student is unable to join in this mainstream use of technology in the classroom, this gap needs to be addressed in order to truly maintain that neutral playing field. If a student is not engaged, they will find ways to see their outsideness. Your job as faculty is to focus on inclusivity, even though not everyone likes the same thing. Not an easy task, but an important one. Perhaps those who do not embrace technology as much can have an equally important role when playing games (such as scorekeeper, referee, or coach). Maybe you can find a game they enjoy and alternate. Whatever it is, it is important to play games that each person can participate in, or at least be part of.

What Did You Use as Your Litmus?

Whether you felt it was a great day, a rough week, or somewhere in between, how did you gauge this? When things are going well, there is a synergy, a connection with your students much like a transcendence. Figuratively, light bulbs of understanding go off, as an "aha, I understand" moment; it is in these moments most faculty find their true enjoyment of teaching. Did you get that connection? Did you expect it? If you expected but did not get it, what else did you use to gauge whether there was a connection? Did students come up and chat with you at the break or after class? Obviously, if they are rushed to the next class or to get to work, there may not be a huge crowd. However, usually one or two students might approach faculty after class and confirm an assignment or ask for clarity, or even simply be social. If they didn't, did you avail yourself to that possibility? Were you approachable, or busily collecting homework and cleaning off the whiteboard? How did you make yourself open to the possibility of being wanted?

What are you using to determine if the day was good or great? How do you know if it was a bust or needed improvement? Are you comparing yourself to others? Why? Are you feeling that you don't have a connection, or that the environment isn't conducive to your style? The great news is that your students have never (unless they are returning) had you before in this class; even if they had a similar class or had you as a teacher before, this is a new opportunity—for you and for them. Every day gives you an opportunity to make it better, keep it fresh, try something different. Only you know what you planned for the day. No one but you will evaluate whether you reached the goals you had planned for the day. The only judge of how the day went is you. Students will have their own perceptions; however, as discussed, their perceptions can be askew. Even if you and your students didn't seem to connect, it is always a good idea to simply ask. Often you may find that they felt the day went well, but may be preoccupied due to a test, work, or home life. They may have enjoyed the day and felt you did a great job—however, you wouldn't know unless you asked. Never judge yourself against other faculty, your own expectations, or even believing you are alone. All faculty must go through a series of trial and error before they feel that connection and can see it for what it is.

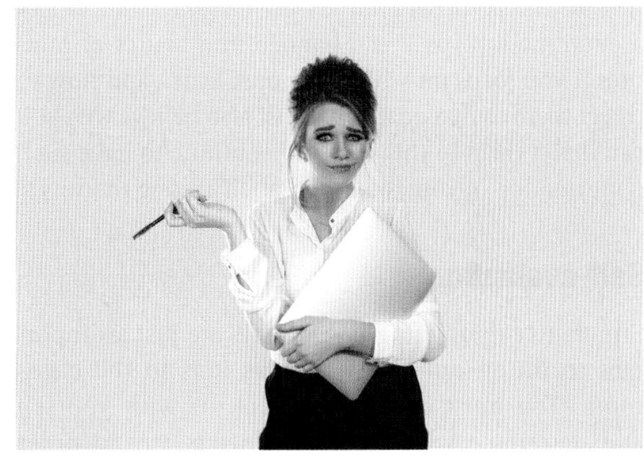

(HbrH/iStock.)

Teaching in a Vacuum

You do not live alone on an island. As such, you do not teach in a vacuum. As stated, you have countless resources, within and outside of yourself. What other jobs have you had? What other skills and talents do you possess? How many other settings have you taught? Even as a parent, a health care provider, or a friend, you have had the chance to show someone else how to do something. How did you know "how" to teach? What other visual aids or references did you use? This information illustrates that when you teach, you use everything and everyone at your disposal to ensure the information gets across to the recipient and that they understand. Think back on a particular task you had to teach someone, or even when you had to help a child with their homework. You got down to the simplest version and went over the material, in short segments, like taking baby steps. You didn't proceed until they got it, and then, slowly, you began to offer a bit more information. Soon they were able to realize that they understood the concept, though it seemed daunting at first. Your patience and persistence gave them the inspiration to continue.

The same is true when teaching multiple students or even multiple classes. You are not expected to do it just with the textbook or PPT slides given to you on a thumb drive. You are expected to think of all the possible resources in the world, on the Internet, within you and within the universe to illustrate the information in such a way that students can understand it. Slowly, in baby steps, in various formats, you bring their awareness to the point where they get it. This is no longer a daunting task, as it can happen in a matter of minutes if you focus on what they must learn, and how to direct them to that goal. You must also believe that you can direct them to this goal and continue to have such confirmation of your skills and ability along the way.

Self-evaluation

Summative or ongoing assessments are just as important to do on our own selves as it is in the classroom. You must constantly check in with yourself and determine what your own needs are, in order to teach, be effective, and not burn out. You must remain objective, maintain focus, and keep your eye on the goals—including the goals you have for your self-care. If you are exhausted, spend less time with your family, and run out of weekend preparing for class, you will most likely find little enjoyment in the long run. You need downtime, time to regroup, refresh, and focus on what you enjoy. You also need time away from students, the campus, and even other teachers. Often when conversing with others outside of education you are able to put things back into perspective, release some negative energy, and perhaps even laugh at yourself (or the circumstances). Remember humor is important; we shouldn't take ourselves too seriously, or even our students. We will serve our students better when we are able to care for ourselves and gain more insight into our humanness. Chapter 2 asked you to pause and reflect on self-care, rest, exercise, and emotional support. Self-TLC can bring new life back into your teaching; it allows you to infuse yourself with new ideas and discover why old ideas didn't work. Other activities that can assist are journaling (hence the reason we have included so much in this chapter), small group discussions (with your peers or others in education), and support groups or blogs. Anytime you bring a group of people with a common interest together you have a chance of bettering the group as they share best practices, mentor one another, and allow for a healthy dose of venting to occur.

As with any profession that cares for others, such as social work, nursing/medicine, counseling, and even retail or customer service jobs, you must learn to give back to yourself. Take time to get out of your rut, go for a walk, do a hobby (or take up a new one), or get involved in another activity. After a night of kickboxing, an afternoon of paintball, or even a quiet evening of reading, you may be able to see your students in a new light. If you don't, perhaps the hobby is not one you enjoy. Make sure that whatever you do during your off time is rewarding and fills the cups of affirmation for you. Teaching is a giving profession; it comes with few accolades and very little acknowledgment for those who may hunger for approval. So, whatever you choose to do to help you feel appreciated, do it frequently.

Martyrdom

Occasionally, faculty may feel that their destiny is teaching, at any cost. They do not focus on self-care, but rather giving to students. Instead of wanting recognition, they defer to their students' talents and expertise. When it comes to offering prizes and rewards, they spend their own time baking, making, and buying treats to make sure students are happy. They don't ask for time off, never request reimbursement, and shy away from any delegation. They take on monumental tasks and feel it is their job to do them all. They spend long hours at the office or on campus, adjust their hours to ensure they meet with students whenever necessary, and feel that they are obligated to meet their students' needs.

While this may seem like benign behavior, it can cause a great deal of friction with other faculty. It can also lead to burnout, low self-esteem, and greater dissatisfaction with your profession. While teaching may be your vocation, and you are fully committed to it, it does not mean that you should practice without boundaries. Indeed, having appropriate boundaries ensures you are doing the best to service your students. It allows you to know when to say no, and when to reexamine your agenda. Are you using students to give you self-satisfaction and secretly need their approval to feel good about yourself? Are you feeling that you must offer selfless service as an act of your faith, or do you believe it is part of your culture? Is this a requirement in order to reap the benefits of the afterworld or do you feel that this is your fate? If you are teaching because you think it is a requirement, and there is no other profession you can do, you may want to reevaluate your interest for entering the profession. You also need to determine what your motivation is, as teaching is often called a labor of love; most teachers don't achieve celebrity status or great wealth, but rather an innate satisfaction that they are doing what they are called to do. Reexamining why you became a teacher, remain a teacher, and how you expect to feel rewarded as a result of this career choice requires a hard look at your motives.

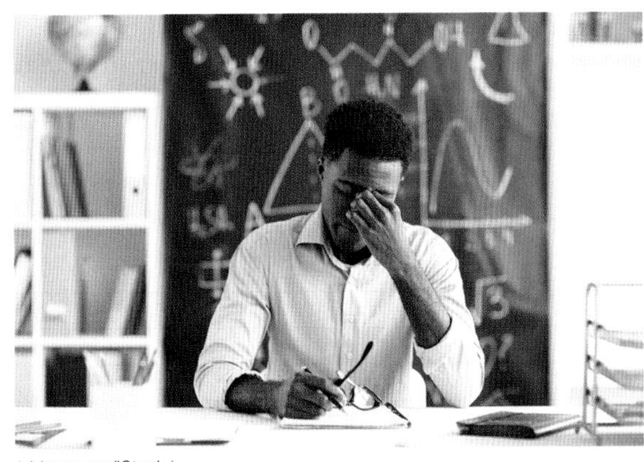

(shironosov/iStock.)

In previous chapters there has been room for journaling, self-reflection, and a chance to ask yourself some questions. Because this chapter is all about you, it is necessary to do more journaling and self-reflection. The exercises below help you connect with yourself, focus on you, and how you will be improving. Our next chapter will focus on developing yourself as a lifelong learner.

Journal: Self-reflection

1 Before we get into your self-assessment and areas to improve, let's look back on previous chapters and determine whether you feel you have learned enough about those topics. In each of the following categories, rate yourself as a beginner, intermediate, advanced, or expert in that specific area. Most people who are new to the teaching profession will be deemed a beginner, which is expected. However, some categories may include prior skills that allow you to feel more of an intermediate or expert. Despite your years of teaching you may still not feel like you know more than the beginner; not to worry—even seasoned teachers may not feel they are an expert in that category.

Category	*Self-rating*
Learning theories	
Course planning	
Classroom management	
Student engagement	
Critical thinking/judgment	
Best practices/effective instruction	
Assessments	
Decreasing the educational gap	

Key: B = Beginner, I = Intermediate, A = Advanced, E = Expert

2 So, you want to be a teacher? This is how we started Chapter 1, and we ask the question again. Do you *still* want to be a teacher? Is this what you had in mind? Share what your vision is or was; what did you envision the day looking like?

3 In reviewing what your class looked like, you have probably come up with a variety of things you felt went right or went wrong. Start jotting down notes of both—things that went well, and those that didn't.

4 In question #3, by whose definition did these things not go right? How did you come to this conclusion?

5 At the end of the day, how did your students react? Did they share how the day went or did you notice their body language? Write down your observations and conversations, if you were able to conduct any.

6 In what ways were you able to assess your students (audience) prior to meeting them? When you did this assessment, where were students in the program (e.g., during orientation, on the first day of class, or another time)?

7 Did you have office hours or time before/after class whereby you could meet with students? How did these meetings go? Did students stop by and ask questions? Did you feel you were able to connect with them, answer their questions, or at least have a conversation? How do you feel about these interactions, or, lack of interactions?

8 How are you feeling overall at this juncture? Write down both positive and negative feelings—don't try to analyze them or determine their origin, just write freely whatever comes to mind.

9 What similarities did you find you had with students? What differences? What about the students among themselves—what are their similarities and differences?

10 In considering your day, how did the classroom environment feel? What was the students' energy like? Did you have any hiccups that were unforeseen? Did you feel that you had some control over the day and the activities?

11 The reference regarding classroom management asked the question whether the monkeys were running the zoo. Did you feel that students were more in charge? Did one or two students seem to monopolize the day or some of the activities? If so, how did that make you feel?

12 What could you have done differently that might have had a more positive impact on your classroom management?

13 Despite the work you put into the day, what did you *not* plan for? As mentioned, there are hiccups in each day.

a. What were yours? What happened that you were not prepared for?

b. In retrospect, how will you address this hiccup in the future? What could you have done differently or will do next time to decrease this hiccup?

14 Student engagement is the crux of active learning. However, it takes time to become proficient and perhaps even comfortable with some of the games, exercises, and activities.

a. What did you like? What did your students like?

b. What did you not like? Or better stated, what did not go over well with your students? What did your students enjoy the most out of your activities?

15 Were there activities you did not feel comfortable doing? What can you do to improve these for next time?

16 Critical thinking exercises are often the most challenging to prepare for and to execute. Which activities went well? Which need more fine tuning?

17 How has your comfort level changed when doing the games, activities, and critical thinking exercises? What resources did you use to gain expertise in delivering these games (Internet, peers, other students, etc.)?

18 In every teacher's experience, there are days that you feel are a total bomb (not in a good way). Have you had one of those days? Share how you felt. If you haven't felt that way, how would you handle it if you ended the day feeling it was a total waste? What might cause you to feel this way?

19 Ongoing assessments are crucial to redirect the faculty member and help you reach the goals, objectives, and ensure you are on course. What assessments did you do? Which ones were most effective?

20 When considering the goals and hitting your mark, where did you fall short? Where was the gap? How about with your students—was there a gap in ages, cultures, or generations? How was your comfort level? What went right or wrong; what was better perceived and what fizzled out? Share a bit more about your experience with this.

21 Based on your experience and your comfort level, what resources do you need? In what areas? List all of those that are available to you on campus, in your community, and among your circle of influences/friends. Who or where else can you go for help?

22 In the next chapter, we will review self-development and lifelong learning. For now, jot down your expectations. What do you feel you need to explore in order to improve?

23 We shared a few of the necessities required to help perform self-care, that TLC you need to prevent burnout. In Chapter 2 you were asked to write down five things you would do to care for yourself—go back and review what you wrote. Have you done these things? Were they effective in helping you feel supported or cared for? If you did not do these five things, or they were not effective, write down why. What other things can you do to help yourself decompress and feel in charge of your career? Write down five more things you will do for self-care.

24 Hobbies, sports, and other recreational activities are a great way to take our minds off our stress and allow our creativity to expand. What activities are you doing/can you do to help you destress? List two that you are using or will try to incorporate this week/month.

____

____

____

____

____

____

Believe you can and you're halfway there
Theodore Roosevelt

Chapter 10

Self-development and Lifelong Learning

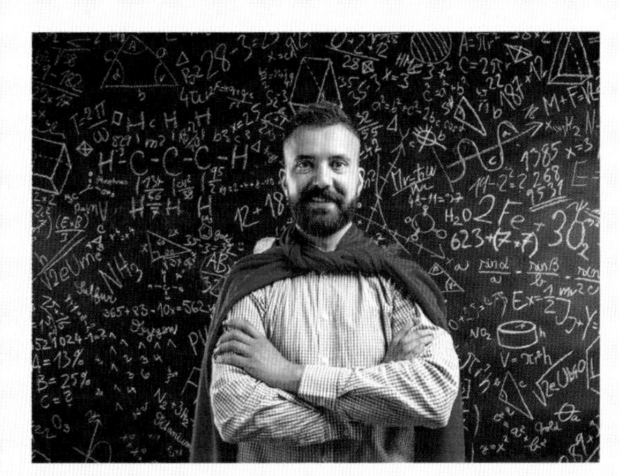

(Halfpoint/iStock.)

I'm a teacher, what's your superpower? Though we often see this saying on various mugs, T-shirts, and other paraphernalia, it is true. As teachers, we can shape the world, the future of all generations, and inspire people to reach their greatest potential. This incredible "superpower" also comes with tremendous responsibility and a powerful accountability. While we are focused on reaching even the most resistant student, we must also keep our eyes on the other students while striving for all students to see the goal, reach the goal, and even surpass the goal. Whether the goal is internal, external, written, or expected, our profession is a lifelong focus on goal setting and acquisition. All of this started with us, and our own desire to reach a goal.

Dreams and Enchantment

Your own career goals were once dreams. You imagined that you could touch another person's life, that you had a lot to give, that the talents you possess were meant to be shared and not hidden. You looked for opportunities and waited ... until one day you got your first teaching job. You fell in love with the idea that you could fashion and mold young minds, that the innocence of youth was alive, and you would have a chance to influence it. You felt that, for the first time in your life, you might be able to make a real difference. You embraced every opportunity to learn more, be more, and, despite how much you learned, you still craved more.

This is not a fairytale idea or a wish that's a shot in the dark. It is not a forgotten hope or a never to be acquired dream. It is real, if it is real to you. And it is attainable, albeit always developing. Being a teacher means you are never stagnant, you are always learning, you are always evolving yourself. Whatever you love about the industry needs to be in the forefront of your mind; it must be your mantra, for there will be days when you feel disenchanted. You may wonder if you missed your mark; it may seem the bad days outnumber the good ones. As you look back on this career, and other careers, there will always be moments you felt that you were on top of the world; there are also other moments you wonder why you chose this profession. Seriously, what were you thinking? You were thinking you could be valued for who you are.

Regardless of whether this is your first teaching job or one of many teaching jobs, you will have days of defeat. You will have days of questioning and days of doubt. You will also have days of triumph, when you watch students walk the stage at graduation, or when a student is asking for a reference. You may have more chances to touch lives as a faculty development specialist, a dean, or simply a peer mentor. Many opportunities will become apparent, but only if you are looking for the positiveness in your profession. Focusing on the good, the triumphs, and the many talents you share can help you when your skepticism prevails.

It can at least keep the cynicism at bay, as you muster up more positive energy to go out and conquer the world. After all, isn't that what you tell your students to do?

What's in Your Way?

When looking at the SMART method (specific, measurable, attainable, realistic, and timely), the first step in goal attainment is believing that you *can* achieve the goal. This includes you—your own belief that you can achieve the goals you desire. If it is simply to be a better teacher, or to teach other subjects, or move up the education career ladder, you must believe in yourself. *You* must have the confidence that you can do the job or acquire the skills necessary to do your job better. It comes down to your own self-efficacy; the same thing you have encouraged in your own students. Do you believe that you are worth a better job, that you can be a better teacher, that you are able to do other jobs within education? Do you have faith that you will be led, or trust the universe to offer these opportunities, or do you feel that it is simply up to you to make it happen? Regardless of your belief system, believing in yourself and your capabilities is paramount. So, what's getting in your way? Usually the only thing getting in your way is you. Let's review your goals again. Considering what you want to do in your profession, think about a few SMART goals. You will have a chance to write about your own goals later in the self-reflection journal. For now, let's review the overall concepts of goals.

Specific

When considering your goals, remember to be specific. As with our example in Chapter 6, it must be so clear that it can be measured by anyone, not just you. One word often (erroneously) used is "better"; though you want to improve, this word defines nothing. To claim you want a "better" job or to know your students "better" doesn't clarify anything. How would anyone know? How could it be measured? A more accurate goal is to have something more tangible, such as an increase in pay, a job at a specific institution, or a particular position. "I want to obtain a full-time job teaching nursing at a vocational program within a community college in New York" is specific. "I want to increase the results of my student surveys from 'x' to 'y' during a specific date period" is specific. Remember, the more detailed, the more opportunity you have to measure and determine if you reached your goal. This can be crucial when considering a career goal, as you also want to let future employers know what you are looking for.

Measurable

If you have done a good job clarifying your goals with very detailed and specific language, it should be easy to measure. In the earlier two examples, if a job becomes available at a 4-year university for an English professor in Wisconsin, you can easily decline it, as it is not anywhere near what you want (never mind that you are not an English major). If you get a call from a talent scout asking if you want to consider a full-time position as an associate professor at a local community college in New York City (NYC), teaching in their licensed practical nurse (LPN) program, you start doing the dance of joy, brush off your CV, and apply immediately. With the second example, if your survey scores result in a 60% satisfaction and your goal was to reach a benchmark (which is at 75%), you realize you still have some work to do when results come in at 70%. Though you improved, you did not reach your goal (it is still worth doing a happy dance, as there was improvement!). It does allow you to reevaluate what else is needed in order for you to reach this benchmark.

Attainable

One of the most important aspects of goal setting is to have attainable, achievable goals. Perhaps you wanted to obtain this job or reach the benchmark in too short of a time period. It could be that you have not learned how to do surveys, or that the areas they want you to improve are not realistic. The job search you want requires that you live in New York and you currently live in Montana. These are examples of goals that are not necessarily attainable right now. However, it does not imply that you cannot attain these goals; it simply means that you must put into place the steps necessary to attain them. It also requires that you reexamine the goals to ensure they are what you want, and what you want right now. Perhaps the job in New York is better served once your children are in college. The 20% spread you desire to achieve in your surveys could be better achieved in smaller chunks, perhaps a 15% increase in satisfaction is acceptable, as it reaches the benchmark. The additional 5% increase you desire could be better attained after you have had a chance to research the areas that students have asked for.

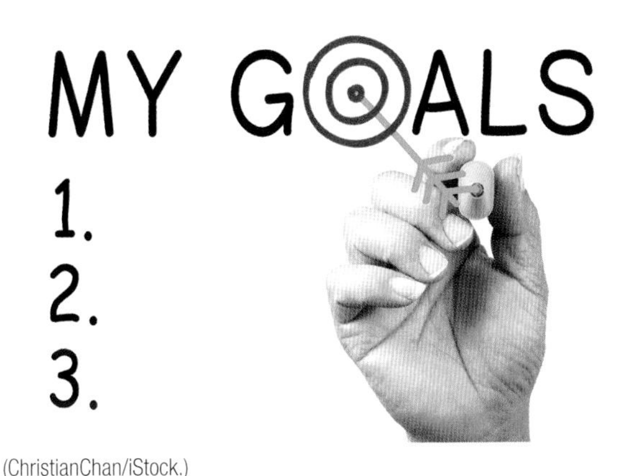

(ChristianChan/iStock.)

Relevant

Your short-term goals need to be relevant to what you are pursuing, but what you are pursuing needs to be relevant to your longer term goals. If you want to be nominated for an award as an outstanding teacher and want this to help you find a new job, it doesn't add up. While being nominated as an outstanding teacher is certainly worthy to post on your résumé or CV, it won't help you get the next job you want. If, however, your goal is to improve as a faculty member, then the nomination is appropriate. When considering your goals, you must look at the details without losing sight of the big picture.

Timely

The most important piece, other than "specific," is the timeframe. To simply state you want a change, without including the timeframe, can leave you frustrated when it doesn't happen. Let's say that you wanted a job in New York within a year. If you did not state that in your goal setting and got depressed after 3 months of searching, you got in your own way. If the survey results increase in slow increments, and you are at 70% after two quarters, you feel that you have made no improvements. However, if you wanted to increase your survey results within the next three quarters, there is still hope. Don't get discouraged—get real. What specifically can you attain within the realistic timeframe? That is the crux of making SMART goals.

Growth and Development

In all humans and living beings, there is an attempt to grow. Life prevails despite the odds; we develop, often without knowing where or how. As a child, a seedling, an egg, or even mountains, there is an inner or an outer movement. We are influenced by our surroundings, the nourishment needed (except for the mountain, though they grow despite the lack of nourishment), and the interaction we have with our environment. As part of our growth and development, we are constantly communing with other sources; we must give and take as we build a relationship within our environment. This is true regardless of what kind of environment we are interacting with; whether nature, a society, a campus, or within ourselves. Each of these environments must allow a chance for us to integrate and assimilate. We provide information, receive information, process information, and adapt. This is how life survives and thus how we must survive as an ongoing species, as a profession, and as a human being. Our job does not end at the completion of a class or at the end of a day. We don't hang up our hat and call in the cavalry and say we're done. Even when we feel that we have given our all, we have more to give. This is the symbiotic connection we have with the world. As a teacher, we thrive to excel, to join forces with like-minded folks, to be a part of something bigger. If we get out of our way, we often can achieve these goals and more, as there is no end to learning. This is what is referred to as lifelong learning. As the directors of the educational flow it is important than we embrace this learning as we pass it on to our students, our managers, and our peers. In doing so, we perpetuate the industry and advocate for more learners and learning.

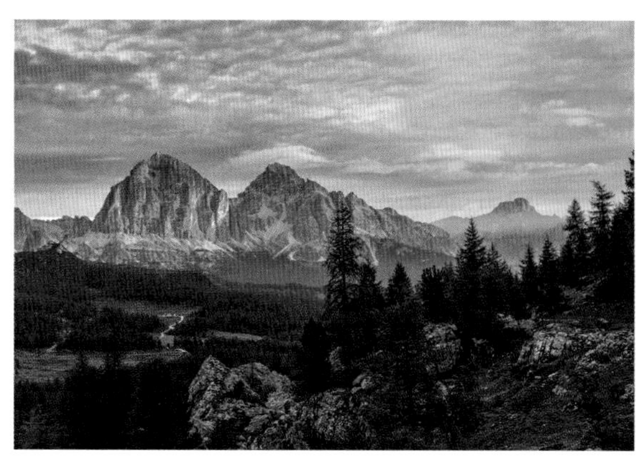

(Elena-studio/iStock.)

Lifelong Learning

Lifelong learning implies we are continuously seeking new information, looking not for finite answers, but actually more questions. We search out more areas that we don't know, ask more questions in an attempt to learn more, and once we know, we feel we know nothing. This is not a bad thing, as it is the motivation that keeps us pursuing how to be a more knowledgeable teacher, well rounded in our quest, seeking to add to our repertoire of information. We are a bottomless pit of data, always pursuing the next great thing that will help us be more effective and able to connect on a deeper level with others, ourselves, and our world. As exciting as this may sound, it is important to also temper this quest with realism. We will never know everything about ourselves or the subject matter we teach. We will never have a finite end to our own learning. There is no acme to reach in the courses despite the many books, articles, and research conducted. Because there are millions of people studying the very same thing we are teaching, our teaching focus is in a microcosm of other learners, teachers, and studies that will influence and change over time. This outcome is a kaleidoscope that is never the same again but will always reveal a new angle. Therefore, despite the years we have studied to earn our degree, credentials, tenure, and status at our institution, we are never done with learning. Much like parenting, learning continues as we grow old, as we move to different communities, even as we pursue other careers. It becomes an integral part of who we are and how we conduct business. In is in the very fabric of the woven cloth that we are cut from and the tapestry we will become part of. For those who are called to the profession of teaching, the lifelong process of learning more is in our blood and propels us to move forward in a never-ending state of learning. There is no goal except to become more whole, more unified, and more complete.

More About You

As you set off and chart your career path for more adventures, where do you want to go? How do you want to be? Who do you want to become? Within your teaching profession, how will you attain these goals? Let's return to why you wanted to be a teacher. How did you come to this place in your career? What do you like or dislike about the profession? Much like the exercises on expectations, you will need to revisit what you want this career to look like, and thus, as a lifelong quest, how you will know when you see it. What more do you want to do? Why? Where will you go to do it?

Let's review your strengths. What strengths are you bringing to the profession of teaching? What innate skills do you already have? It can be soft skills, such as verbal communication (perhaps you are a great storyteller or orator); maybe you help people feel at ease and are great with customer service. It could be that you have a knack for explaining things in a way people understand. These skills are very important in numerous professionals, especially in teaching. If you had other jobs prior to this one, what transferable skills do you have? Were you a leader in your industry? Did you work closely on intense projects with strict deadlines? Are you more of a solitary worker or a team builder? How much do you enjoy following protocols and policies? Are you a stickler for such protocols or more of a free-spirited person? Each of these qualities can benefit you as a teacher as well as help you obtain other jobs in education. Being that the student is our customer, we strive to ensure their needs are met. While they may not always be satisfied, they should be able to satisfy their goals. Our ability to work with others is necessary in teaching; it is also often a skill we bring to the profession. Previous careers easily dovetail into teaching and can guide us as we learn more about ourselves and try to test the water toward new growth.

Your Vocation

Teaching is a career as well as a vocation. If you stumbled upon this accidently, you need to reevaluate the same as if this had been your lifelong dream. Is teaching what you want to do, or what you see yourself doing 20 years from now, and is it in alignment with what your aptitude is? This is a crucial question as it will direct you as you find what your next step is, if there is really a next step. There are several books in circulation, as well as on the Internet, regarding how to select the best career path, how to assess your aptitudes, personality type, and values. The important thing is that there is a connection; whether you feel it slightly or tightly, you know that this is what you want to do. Such a sense of assurance brings confidence in times of despair and can rekindle the motivation to keep you on the track of learning. Whether you see it as a calling from a higher power, a moral sense of responsibility, a higher caste, or simply what you love doing, the impetus behind your choice to be a teacher may need to be reviewed from time to time. There is always room for additional self-discovery; further opportunities to explore, and deeper knowledge to acquire when considering self.

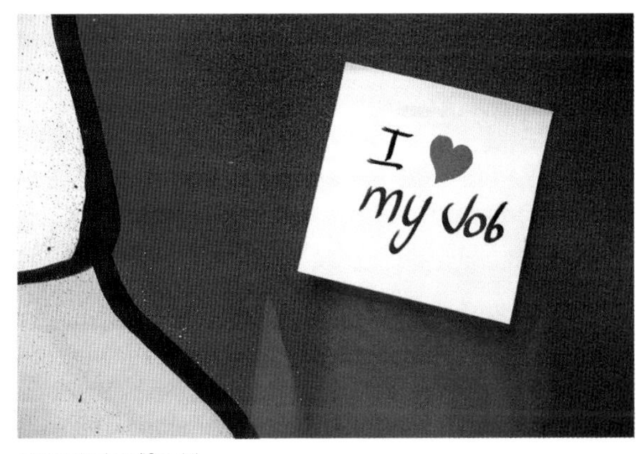

(studiostockart/iStock.)

While many of the chapters focused on how we teach others, we must also understand how we learn and to teach ourselves. As we continue this cycle, we will find innumerable chances to grow and develop. We will be better equipped to know our self, our desires, and be able to satisfy them in a way that keeps us wanting more. As with our students, we can become satiated but never fully satisfied. Once again, lifelong learning does not occur overnight; hence the words "life" and "long." As long as you are alive, you are learning.

Busyness

What have you decided you like about teaching? Maybe you have not spent time thinking too much about it as you are too busy learning the profession right now. There is something to be said for being busy, as it keeps our focus on something other than what we want to do (or should be doing). Often, we are so busy we forget to do the simplest things, like eat healthy (or eat at all), exercise, or spend quality time with family. We are enthralled in our lesson plans, our activities, meeting with peers, students, and other departments and we lose sight of our growth. Some people think that if they are not busy, they are not productive. If they are idle, they are stagnant and not productive. What is often missed is that in quiet times, we allow change to occur. Stillness invites such quiet, where silence welcomes deep growth and transformation. Instead of seeing such idleness as a negative thing we can take the chance to sit quietly with our self, or with others. We can start communing instead of filling our time with communication. We email, call, text, have meetings, webinars, and training on myriad topics but fail to simply stop and listen to our inner beings. When considering our vocation, personal growth, and development, as well as our future, we must allow time to digest, rest, and refill our empty cups of energy. We must be still and in step with nature or whatever we connect with. In these moments, we often find the guidance we are seeking and this brings us greater satisfaction. These infusions of life are necessary to keep us on track, prevent burnout, and allow us to focus on the betterment of our profession and vocation.

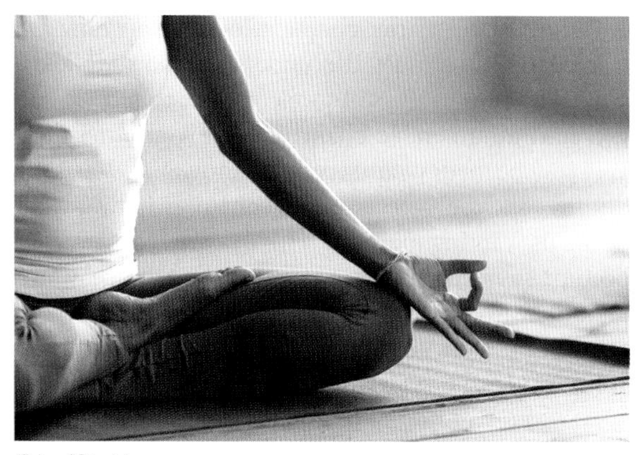

(fizkes/iStock.)

What's Next

So, what does your future look like? As the adage says, "What do you want to do when you grow up?" If this is your first time teaching a class, what other classes are you interested in teaching? There will be several journal entries to help you brainstorm as your innermost desires remain with you, even if the course changes from time to time. Consider this example of a teacher who wanted to be an engineer. However, her culture did not approve of a woman being in a predominantly male-focused profession. As a young woman, she got married and started a family. Although her husband was supportive of her interest, they decided it was best for her to be at home with the children. She put her goals of education on hold until the children were old enough to start school, and then she investigated various programs. When she met with the guidance counselor at the local community college, she did several aptitude tests and personality profiles. The results came back with a list of various professions, one of which was teaching. This was a field she had not considered but began looking into. She felt she didn't have the right qualities to be a teacher, despite the various tests. However, she brought the material home and began to research what teachers did and what attributes they had. After pursuing the material, she realized that her desire to be an engineer stemmed from her knack for seeing the big picture, extrapolating data, and understanding detailed calculations. She was excellent in math and could explain things in a simplified version, a tactic she used frequently on her children when she helped them with their homework. She later returned to the community college and began taking courses in education. As she earned her first degree, she realized that many of the talents that she thought would be used in engineering could be used in the classroom setting. She taught basic subjects in math, science, and related disciplines. After 10 years of teaching she chose to earn her second degree; this time, in mathematics. She moved on to the 4-year college and started teaching in the business department and focused on the engineering cohorts. She was able to use her skills in teaching math, her role as mother, and her passion for engineering to guide new freshmen to their first courses in college. Though she later went on to obtain her terminal degree in engineering, she realized that had she started with that degree, she never would have found the fulfillment of teaching or her love of other subjects, mainly math.

Before you go on to the next level, you must decide what you want to do now. However, you may not be ready to make it too specific. It could be that you want to maintain where you are for a few years—then move on to a higher degree or teach in a different setting. You may want to branch out or you may want to wait until you feel comfortable. Of course, when you're ready to create your SMART goals, you'll need to ensure there is some concrete pathway, even if (as in our above example) the path goes along a different course than you originally thought.

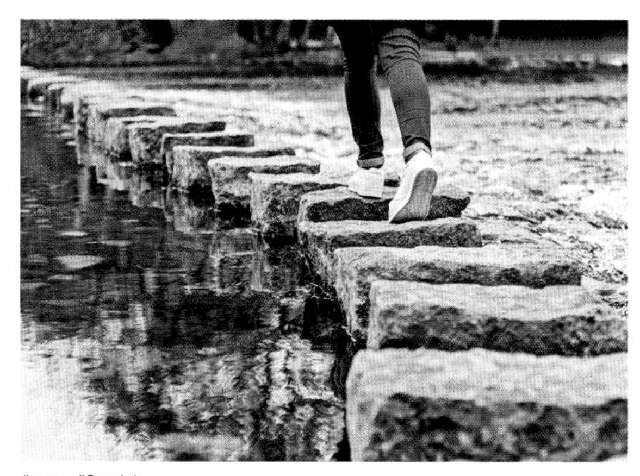

(baona/iStock.)

How to Achieve the Next Level

Considering all this, what *is* the next level for you? How will you get there? Do you need more experience, or another degree, or an interim position? When we consider that we are lifelong learners, we also need to include the fact that we are constantly expanding our comfort zone. Although we have our current job, our career, our degrees/education, and experiences, we need to add more to our repertoire in order to move on. Move on to what? This is the question we will continue to ask ourselves along the way may times over. What does the next level, or moving on, look like? Who do I need to add to my circle of influence to help me get there? What else is required in order to achieve the next level? Who can help me? Using the Socratic method works well in this situation as much as it does in our classroom; as Socrates would have us recall, the answers are within us. The point is to discover more about ourselves, so we find the answers. Lifelong learning commits to an unquenchable desire to learn more. But what does "more" look like?

Continuously Improving

In many service industries, as well as health care, we look at quality control. We want to use services and products efficiently and ensure that they are rendered the best. The same is true in education; we are always striving to do our best. We ask this of our students, our institutions, our clinical facilities, our externships sites, and of ourselves. We try to "do better," we look at results and attempt to advance to a higher status, a more superior outcome. To be the "best" implies we have utilized all measures to do what no one else has really done. In our own world, it could mean that we want to teach more effectively, increase our ability to connect with students and engage them further; perhaps we need to acquire more effective classroom management skills to do this. Continuously improving could imply that we expand our weak areas, subjects that are not our strengths, or facets of teaching we remain a novice at. All of this occurs at various levels in teaching, as we never arrive at the "destination" but are always on the journey.

The Journey

Every journey starts with one step. You have at least taken that first step. What steps you take afterward are up to you. However, a few things are known: you won't go any further without continuing to take steps; each step brings you closer to where you want to go or where you want to be; stepping takes time, it is not a jump or a catapult, it is simply a step. All steps are to lead you somewhere, and are usually over something: a bridge, a river, a staircase, up a ladder (over something), or some other obstacle. The point is, do you have the stamina to go over whatever that obstacle is, to take the next step? In order to answer this question, you must again, go back inside yourself.

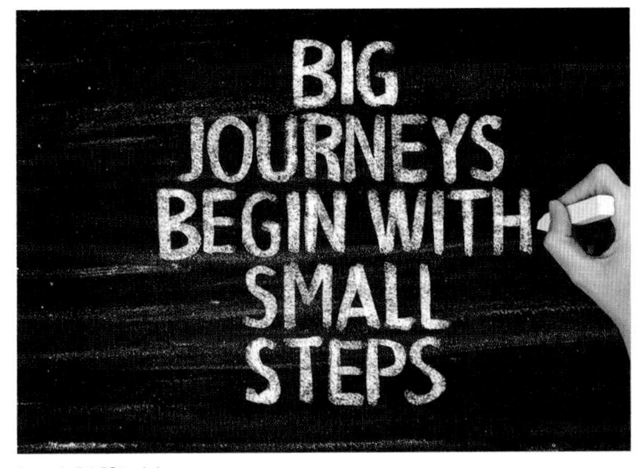

(marrio31/iStock.)

Self-discovery

It seems elementary that we go back to our own dreams of what we "should" be, or what we thought we would become. However, as childish as it seems, these youthful aspirations are necessary to help us understand our own desires. Understanding "self" leaves us in a place of discovery, a perpetual learning in a vastness of the unknown, back to the first place where we chose to enter, a place where we have come from, parched and empty, wanting to receive nourishment and fulfillment. To do this we must go back to our own self, back to the quiet, the solace, the dreams.

What are you made of? Not to sound too schizophrenic, but we all hear voices that help guide us.

Some people consider these voices a sense of direction from the universe, or a higher power. Whether you consider it God, Allah, or your better judgment, those voices often nudge us to improve and can steer us in a healthy course. What is within you that cries out for more, that voice which asks you "are you where you need to be?" What do you hear when you ask what the next steps are? What obstacles are present? In addition to these positive voices, there are probably negative voices as well. These voices may tell you that you can't do it, you are not good enough, or you don't have what it takes. Just as with your students, you too must choose to downplay these negative influences and realize you do have what it takes and are absolutely good enough! Listening to more positive voices, whether inside your head, from your family, or in a work setting, or even from your community or with friends, can have a significant impact on your overall mental health. Often we must realize the contributions we have made and the good things we have accomplished. While we may not have done everything right, we have given it the right focus. And we can look at other goals to see how to succeed with them as well.

Look back on what you have done. Look forward to what you want to do. Where is that gap? Acknowledging that gap will help you realize where you are and where you want to go. It can also help in understanding where you have been and how that relates to your future, based on your next steps. Reflection, as you have done in this book, can be looked back upon to remind yourself of how much you have grown. While you may not have realized it, you have grown since the first chapter, indeed you know more now than you did that first day. The same will be true a few month or years from now; you will reflect on the many accomplishments you have made in your teaching career. To give you a bit of a boost, there are several questions at the end of this chapter that will ask you to consider how much more you know now than when you first began this course. Once again, several questions at the end of this chapter will allow you to savor the moments of growth and see how much progress you have made. Tactics such as reflection are helpful along the way in any profession, but especially in ones where you give a great deal of yourself. Knowing where you are today is part of developing one's self, as it focuses on the present.

Mindfulness

In addition to reflection, we must be mindful of where we are now, today, in this moment. Mindfulness is exactly doing that—being aware of where you are right now. It's not about evaluating your present state or making any judgments about where you are or what you are doing, but simply acknowledging the here and now. This concentrated act allows us to fully and deeply be in the only place where we have any control: the present. The past and future cannot be controlled, and thus we must accept what has been done or will be done. We can learn, adjust, and change our present, but we cannot erase the past, nor can we change it or predict the future. Considering where you are now, being mindful, can be compelling, as it brings into the light all the factors that are happening. Maybe you got off course or took too much on. Perhaps you are right where you belong but have given too much and are fatigued. It could be that this is not what you wanted or has missed the mark slightly. Being mindful can allow you permission to take time and adjust. Your satisfaction is important; your ability to feel confident is crucial; connection on some level with your students is paramount. Mindfulness also allows the feelings and emotions you have to emerge and be recognized. This can be fruitful as you come into better connection with yourself and what you need out of your profession. That connection, coupled with the positive voices, can lead to a very prosperous and enriching vocation!

De-stressing

In addition to mindfulness, other forms of meditation, such as yoga and spiritual practices, can decrease stress. More conventional methods, such as exercise, therapy, and self-help groups can assist. Contemporary practice includes pet therapy (have you ever petted a turkey?), unplugging (can you not respond to any email or text for 24 hours?), and taking on a new hobby (now is the time to practice your air guitar!); all of which simply get you out of yourself and allow the mind to disconnect. While you may see these things as time consuming (a commodity you simply do not have right now), they are an investment. If you don't take time for self-care, chances are you will burn out and not be of any help to your students. You can also be quite cranky (or snarky), feel overextended, and have all your efforts backfire. This obviously does not help you move forward or develop more effective skills to help your students. Being your best, allowing yourself to say "no," and establishing a healthy work–life balance also models to your students how to do the same. You become a great example of how to have a prosperous and rewarding profession, but still have time for yourself and your family. Many times, students need such an example as they may be the first in their family to attend college and may not have a role model to guide them. Establishing healthy practices also influences your peers, who may also be overextending themselves or not using good time management skills. We all have 24 hours in a day. How we use them is up to us; if we had more time in the day most of us would fill it up with more tasks to do. Staying focused on what we must do and ensuring we get the most urgent needs of any day taken care of (including ourselves) are good habits to have.

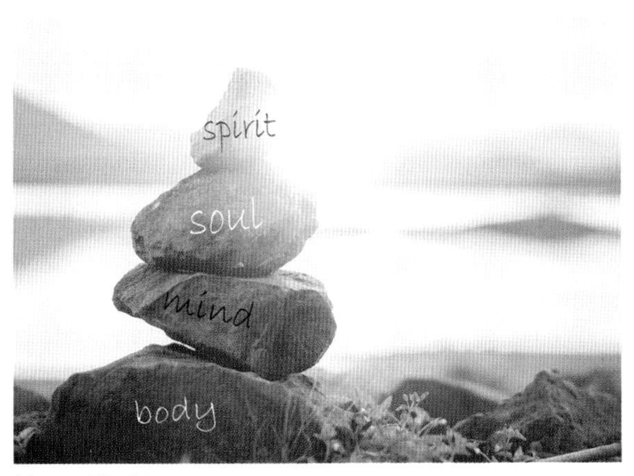

(Urupong/iStock.)

In Chapter 3, you wrote your own serenity prayer. Have you said it, copied it, and posted it in your home or office? Do you take time to simply be quiet or allow that serenity to infuse your space? You have also written words of encouragement over the previous nine chapters. Have you reread them, or taken them to heart? Don't discount how powerful your own words are to you; they are written by the one person who knows you the best: *you*. Believe in you and count your positive words of encouragement as part of your daily routine. You will thank your own self.

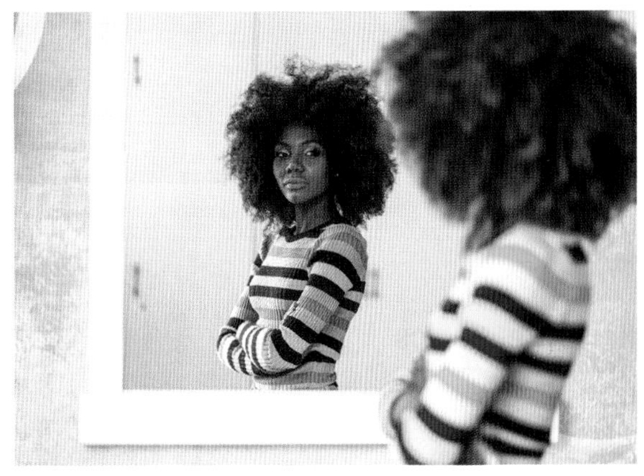

(valentinrussanov/iStock.)

Needs

In Chapter 1 we looked at Maslow's hierarchy of needs. Where are your needs right now? Which level on the pyramid are you? Have things changed since you started teaching? What could help you get to the next level on the pyramid?

These needs are important, as each level needs to be fulfilled, even if you are searching for self-actualization or transcendence (review Chapter 1 on this idea). You must also include how your institution or other resources are assisting you in your needs when it comes to resources. Have you spent time with your mentor reviewing the material? Do you feel that you have enough knowledge to know what resources are at your disposal in the classroom with regard to your institution? If not, make sure you bring this up. It is their goal to have all employees orientated and up to speed, but they, too may be challenged with time restraints. Don't expect that they already know what you need—respectfully speak up and share any other resources you are unclear about, or unsure if they are offered.

Maslow's hierarchy of needs

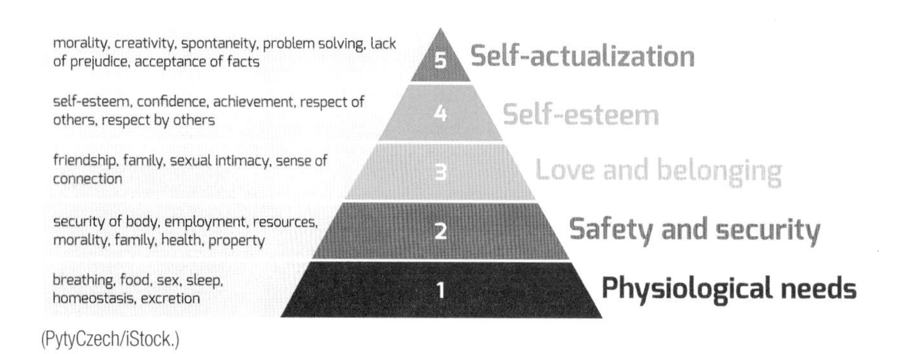

(PytyCzech/iStock.)

Review of Basics

As we have spent a great deal of time reflecting, we must also look at some of the specifics from the beginning to ensure we have a solid foundation to build upon. For starters, are you competent with understanding the various learning theories and how each one can influence your teaching? It could be fruitful to review your reflection on what activities you stated you would use in the classroom. Did one theory speak to you louder when you went to execute it in the classroom? Perhaps you would like to learn more about that theory and how to master it, even the Socratic method. Gardner's multiple intelligences theory (MIT) opened many opportunities for you to explore, both with your students and within your subject matter. How did those classes go? Do you feel like a novice with your own learning style? Have you tried other learning styles and used them—with success? If you did not feel that they were successful, what could you do differently? Bloom's taxonomy goes over the basic classification of learning; it is often referred to as the crux of education. How comfortable are you with this taxonomy—did you use it, refer to it, or have a clear understanding of what it means? If not, be sure to speak with your mentor about this or search for more about it on the Internet. You will appreciate how much direction you can glean from these levels.

Fail or Pass?

Obviously, this course is neither a pass nor fail course. However, you are the evaluator. Did you feel that you have passed the exercise with a good understanding of what you need? If you feel as if you need more expertise in certain areas, review them again. You will have an opportunity to reflect further and hopefully speak with your mentor or a manger about areas you want to improve on and the resources you will need to help you. Only you know if you are doing well, have a clue, or still feel completely lost. And unfortunately, you are also the only one to direct yourself to the proper resources to help you.

What else can help you feel that you are making a difference? How else do you need to motivate or inspire yourself? The reflection questions that follow will continue to guide you, and as you understand more about yourself, you will realize better what you bring to the profession. Along the path of your career, you will continue to self-evaluate and adapt, and hopefully look back and realize how much you have shared of yourself and in the lives of others. As you go about your day, always remember your superpowers.

Journal: Self-reflection

1. Starting with the beginning, what was your dream about being a teacher?

2. How have those dreams been nourished or shot down? Do you feel enchanted or disenchanted?

3. How can you fall back in love with the idea of teaching? Or if you feel you are still in love, how will you nurture those feelings?

4 What has challenged you or got in your way of those dreams?

5 Though you cannot prevent these obstacles from getting in your way again, how will you notice if other things are trying to obscure your vision/dreams in teaching?

6 What will you do about such obstacles or distractions? Where can you go to help you get back on course and stay on track?

7 What continues to motivate or inspire you?

8 As previously mentioned, you bring a variety of skills to the profession, such as prior work experience, soft skills, and other non-teaching skills. Elaborate on these skills (share at least five).

9 To get to the next level, you must be clear on what you want and how to get there. What "level" do you want (such as a higher degree, more classes, or …) to reach?

10 What will it take to get to this next level?

11 What resources do you have or need to reach this next level?

12 Do you believe that you are a lifelong learner? What does this mean to you?

13 List two SMART goals as you consider your future as a lifelong learner, or to help you become more of a lifelong learner (note: these are different than the goals mentioned in Chapter 6).

a. Goal #1:

S ____________________

M ____________________

A ____________________

R ____________________

T ____________________

Notes on this goal:

____

____

____

____

b. Goal #2:

S ____________________

M ____________________

A ____________________

R ____________________

T ____________________

Notes on this goal:

____

____

____

____

14 Quiet time and solitude can often be hard to include in your busy life, yet they can also be very powerful times. What "busyness" currently captures your attention?

____

____

____

____

____

15 What time do you have for quiet and solitude? Where do you go to be quiet and still? How often do you go there?

____

____

____

____

____

____

16 What measures have been effective for you to de-stress? List at least two that are currently effective and two new ones you will try.

17 What are your thoughts of mindfulness? What does this look like for you? Are you able to stay in the present? How?

18 When you wrote your serenity prayer, did you use it, or perhaps felt it didn't "speak" to you? Perhaps you need to refresh it, after having some experience teaching. In the space provided, write down your new prayer, mantra, or positive encouragement so that it fits better for where you are in your teaching profession.

19 In this chapter, we referred to the "voices" in our head, both those that are positive and those that are negative. Share a bit more about where these voices come from, and which ones are positive and those that are negative. What do they say? Remember—be as specific as you can, this is for your reflection only.

20 Considering these voices, there are many positive things that you have done since you started teaching. Whether you are new to the profession or are continuing down a great path, you have given much to your vocation. List at least five positive things you have contributed since you started this journey (if you have taught previously, you may include a few, but try to focus on the most recent contributions you have made).

21 In light of all that you have done, what do you still need to improve? As a lifelong learner and focusing on continuous improvement, what else do you strive for to be a better teacher?

22 If you were to give yourself a grade for this course, what would it be? Why?

23 What would you do differently if you had the chance to do this course again or to orientate again?

24 What would you say to yourself or to another new employee to help them succeed in their first few months?

25 What have you enjoyed most about this short journey into the world of teaching? What have you enjoyed the least? Why?

26 "I teach, what's your superpower?" Make this your new mantra! In the space below, list all of your superpowers as a teacher.

Believe in yourself! Have faith in your abilities!
Without a humble but reasonable confidence
in your own powers you cannot be successful or happy.
Norman Vincent Peale

Index

Page numbers followed by 't' indicate tables.

H

I

J

K

L

M

N

O

P

Q

R

S

T

V

W

Y

Z